Wound Care at End of Life

A Guide for Hospice Professionals

Kyna Setsor Collier, RN, BSN, CHPN
Clinical Nurse Educator, HospiScript Services

Bridget McCrate Protus, RPh, PharmD, CGP, MLIS
Director of Drug Information, HospiScript Services

Connie L. Bohn, RN, BSN, CWON
Wound, Ostomy & Continence Nurse, The Ohio State University Wexner Medical Center

Jason M. Kimbrel, RPh, PharmD, BCPS
Vice President of Clinical Services, HospiScript Services

HospiScript Services, a Catamaran Company

HospiScript Services, a Catamaran Company
4525 Executive Park Drive
Montgomery, AL 36166
Tel: 866-970-7500
www.hospiscript.com

ISBN-10: 0-9889558-2-2
ISBN-13: 978-0-9889558-2-0

Acknowledgements:

Charles W. Mason, DO – Reviewer/Collaborator

Board Certified Am Os Bd Family Practice; Hospice & Palliative Medicine

Assistant Medical Director, HomeReach Hospice

To the Staff of HospiScript Services:

The authors wish to thank all of our colleagues for their assistance in the creation of this resource. Without their generous support this work would not have been possible. Their compassionate commitment to improving end of life care for all individuals is an inspiration.

This book provides guidance for the assessment and palliative management of wounds.
Many factors influence whether healing a wound is a realistic goal. Whether the goal is for healing or for symptom relief, untreated wounds can lead to physical discomfort and impair quality of life. It is necessary that they receive appropriate intervention.

How to Use This Book:

Wound Care at End of Life is intended to be a quick reference guide for palliative management of wounds in hospice care. The authors and collaborators have systematically reviewed and collected the pertinent literature and resources related to palliative wound care.

- For those already skilled in wound care, this book can become a resource for support of current practices and a quick treatment lookup tool.
- For those with less wound care experience, this book can become a learning guide and a resource to ensure that all modalities of wound care are addressed during patient care visits.
- For educators, this book may be used as a training guide to address the basics of palliative wound care and assist learners in developing a comprehensive plan of care for the patient with wounds.

Table of Contents

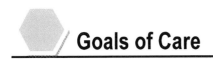 **Goals of Care**

GOALS OF CARE:

The goal of palliative care is symptom control that promotes comfort and quality of life by addressing individual physical, psychological, social and spiritual needs. This same goal applies to palliative wound care, when patients at end-of-life have wounds that may or may not heal.

"The skin is essentially a window into the health of the body"
Sibbald, Krasner, Lutz: SCALE[1]

Wounds are a symptom of advanced disease processes and co-morbidities. Products designed to heal acute wounds may not have the same effect on chronic, non-healing wounds or in patients with poor nutritional intake. However, a patient's quality of life can be improved or at least maintained by controlling symptoms, such as pain, exudate, infection, odor, and bleeding. Patients and caregivers should be able to focus on activities that are important to them. Wound care decisions must be made with patient goals in mind and will be influenced by the location of care and disease progression, as well as other priorities of the patient and family.

"Comfort may be the overriding and acceptable goal, even though it may be in conflict with best skin care practice"
Sibbald, Krasner, Lutz: SCALE[1]

Goals of care may be developed relative to the likelihood of healing the wound.[1,2]
- Wound is healable within the patient's life expectancy
- Wound may be maintained without progression
- Wound is non-healable or palliative care is desired

Treatment plans consistent with patient and family goals of care depend on:[1,2]
- Accurate wound diagnosis
- Patient life expectancy and wishes
- Family member expectations and capabilities
- Institutional policies at the patient's residential care facility

BUILDing the Goals of Care

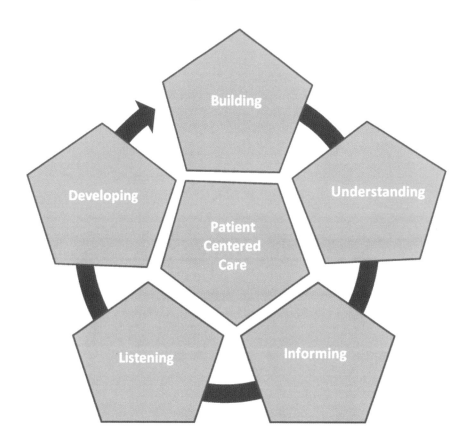

Developing Goals of Care Using the BUILD™ Model		
Component	**Description**	**Key Conversation Points & Phrases**
BUILD the foundation	Build trust and respect	• "Thank you for talking with me today" • "I appreciate you sharing your thoughts with me" • "This must be very difficult for you" • "Are you ready to talk about this?"
UNDERSTAND the patient	Understand how the wound impacts the patient and family	• "What are you hoping hospice can do for you?" • "Help me understand what you'd like to see happen" • "I want to make sure we're on the same page" • "How can I be of help today?" • "Tell me what you understand about your wound right now"
INFORM the patient	Provide information on wound treatment and expected outcomes	• Wound treatment risks and benefits • Disease progression • Role of the hospice team members
LISTEN to the patient	Listen as the patient shares wound care goals; use active listening techniques	• "How is this wound impacting your quality of life?" • "How is wound care impacting your quality of life?" • "Tell me what you are noticing about your wound" • "What wound treatments have or have not been helpful?"
DEVELOP a plan with the patient	Develop a plan of care including the patient, family, hospice, and patient's circle of caregivers	• Negotiate treatment plan • "This is a process, not an event" • Acknowledge the patient/family as decision-makers • Agree to disagree • Revisit the topic on an ongoing basis

BUILDing the Goals of Care

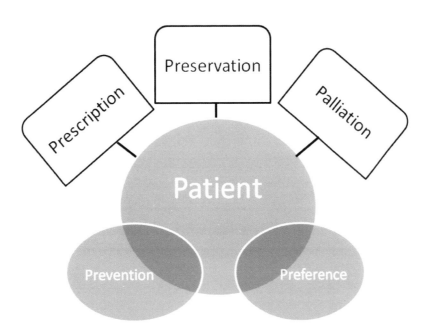

Regardless of determined goal, Prevention and patient Preference are ALWAYS included in care plan:

Prescription: Goal is healing wound with appropriate treatment. Care plan includes interventions for treatable wounds. Even at end-of-life, some wounds may be healable with appropriate treatments. Interventions must:
   • Treat the cause
   • Remain patient-centered
   • Address quality of life concerns (eg: pain, odor)

Preservation: Goal is stabilizing wound condition; healing is unlikely, but deterioration is preventable with appropriate treatment. Care plan recognizes that wound healing or improvement is limited; maintenance becomes the desired outcome. The wound may have the potential to heal but overriding factors (eg: patient refuses treatment, caregiver limitations, inadequate nutrition) result in preservation as the care plan goal.
Palliation: Goal is comfort and symptom management; healing is not possible and wound may deteriorate even with best care. Care plan focuses on patient comfort, not healing, and acknowledges that wounds may deteriorate due to disease progression or dying process. Patients with palliative wound care goals may benefit from modest interventions (eg: autolytic or enzymatic debridement, support surfaces).
Prevention: Care plans should address excessive pressure, friction, shear, moisture, nutrition, and patient mobility. See following sections on environmental, physiologic factors, and support surfaces.
Preference: Preference considers the preferences of the patient and the patient's caregivers. For example, the patient may choose "position of comfort" resulting in greater potential for skin breakdown.
Adapted from SCALE: Skin Changes at Life's End[1]

Chapter 1 References

1. Sibbald RG, Krasner DL, Lutz J. SCALE: Skin changes at life's end: final consensus statement: October 1, 2009. *Adv Skin Wound Care* 2010;23(5):225-236
2. Krasner DL, Rodeheaver GT, Sibbald RG. Interprofessional wound caring. In Krasner DL, Rodeheaver GT, Sibbald RG, eds. *Chronic Wound Care: A Clinical Sourcebook for Healthcare Professionals.* 4th ed. Malvern, PA: HMP Communications. ©2007, p.3-9

EDUCATION:

Evidence-based medicine is a requirement for wound care. Clinicians are demanding evidence before changing a wound care regimen or introducing new products. Evidence-based wound practice is "the integration of best research evidence with clinical expertise and patient values."[1]

Lack of knowledge is one of the most common barriers associated with a failed plan of care. Pressure ulcer incidence increases if clinician knowledge is insufficient. Clinician training should be repeated at regular intervals to address both staff changes and guideline modifications.[2] The clinician must assume responsibility for self-education and recognize it is not a one-time event. Best education practices also help patients and families formulate realistic expectations about their wound treatments, risks, and healing.

Patient education begins with an assessment of the patient's knowledge base and then BUILDing on this foundation. Just as BUILDing the goals of care are patient-centered, education must also be patient-centered. Printed materials are time-savers; however when developing them, carefully consider patient/caregiver educational level, health literacy, cultural and language sensitivities.[3] BUILD on the patient and caregiver's knowledge of the wound and wound care. Take into consideration the emotional and psychological impact the wound has on the patient and family. Wound pain, odor, and exudate have the potential to cause significant social isolation and embarrassment for both the patient and the family. Often, wound care falls to a single caregiver, which may result in that caregiver feeling isolated. If the wound deteriorates, the caregiver may be criticized by other family members even though the deterioration is related to disease process rather than inadequate care. Patients are often embarrassed by the odor, leakage of fluid from the wound, and the unpleasant appearance of the wound. Consciously or subconsciously, wounds are often perceived as a failure on the part of patient or caregiver to provide adequate care. The wound may be perceived as a betrayal by one's own body. The wound is a constant reminder of the presence of disease and the dis-ease it creates.

Provide education for the patient and the patient's circle of care. This may include family, caregivers in the home, or care facility staff (e.g., extended care facilities or assisted living facilities). Hospice interdisciplinary team members may facilitate communication, assist in collaboration, and provide education in managing the patient's skin care needs.

Chapter 2 References
1. Sibbald RG, Woo K, Ayello E. Increased bacterial burden and infection: NERDS and STONES. *Adv Skin Wound Care* 2006:19(8):447-461
2. Ayello EA, Capitulo KL, Fowler E, Krasner DL, Mulder G, Sibbald RG, Yankowsky KW. Legal issues in the care of pressure ulcer patients: key concepts for health care providers: a consensus paper from the International Expert Wound Care Advisory Panel. *J Palliat Med* 2009;12(11):995-1008
3. Nix DP, Peirce B. Noncompliance, nonadherence, or barriers to a sustainable plan? In Bryant RA, Nix DP, eds. *Acute & Chronic Wounds: Current Management Concepts.* 4th ed. St Louis, MO:Elsevier/Mosby. © 2012, p408-415

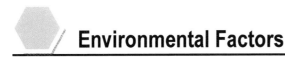

ENVIRONMENTAL FACTORS:

Successful treatment of a wound requires a holistic approach incorporating assessment of the entire patient and co-existing environmental factors, not just the wound. This comprehensive approach identifies and then controls or eliminates factors that impact wound healing. Environmental factors include offloading pressure, providing the appropriate support surface, protecting the skin from moisture, and reducing shear and friction. Develop wound care plans in conjunction with the patient and caregiver, determining what causes them the most concern, seeking their input in developing a plan of care.

Minimize Pressure:

Patient immobility is the most significant risk factor in pressure ulcer development.[1] Offloading pressure creates an environment that enhances soft tissue viability and promotes healing of pressure ulcers. Support surfaces alone neither prevent nor heal ulcers. They are part of the total program of prevention and treatment. Other interventions to offload pressure include:[2]

- *Repositioning*: Shift and adjust patient position at least every 2 hours if at risk for skin breakdown or if skin breakdown is already present. Pillows or foam wedges keep bony prominences from direct contact with one another. Always assess and treat for pain if repositioning causes discomfort to the patient.
- *Pressure relief for heels*: "Floating the heels" is achieved by placing a pillow longitudinally under the calves of the bedbound patient keeping the heels suspended in air. Heel protection devices that completely float the heel are also effective. While no one product has been found to be superior to another, "moon boots" (heel pillows) are not recommended.
- *Side-lying position:* When the patient is positioned on his side, avoid positioning directly on the trochanter.
- *Position of head of bed*: Maintain head of the bed at the lowest degree of elevation medically necessary in order to minimize shear and friction.
- *Lifting devices:* Use of lift sheets will minimize sheer and friction when repositioning the patient.
- *Pressure from sitting:* At risk patients should move at least every hour. If possible, the patient should be taught to shift weight every 15 minutes.
- *Pressure-reducing devices for chairs*: Chair cushions will redistribute pressure. Do NOT use donut-type devices; these tend to cause damage rather than good pressure reduction.

Manage Moisture:

Skin may be exposed to a variety of substances that are detrimental to healing or increase the risk of breakdown due to moisture (e.g., urine, stool, perspiration, wound exudate). The prolonged presence of moisture on the skin places the skin at risk of maceration. Maceration weakens collagen fibers and skin resilience, especially in the presence of mechanical (e.g., friction, tape removal, pressure) or chemical exposure (e.g., harsh skin cleansers, GI secretions, stool).[3] Wet or moist skin has increased fragility, decreased ability to withstand friction and shear, and a tendency to adhere to bed linens. Susceptibility to irritation, rashes, and infection is also increased.[4]

While moisture itself (urine, perspiration, wound exudate) is not caustic to the skin, chemical moisture is caustic due to acidic pH or presence of enzymes.[3] Patients with fecal incontinence are 22 times more likely to develop pressure ulcers than patients who are not incontinent of stool.[5] If moisture or moisture source cannot be controlled, protective barriers and moisture-absorbing products are recommended. See Topical Medicated Agents chart on page 46 for more information.

If the patient is incontinent of urine and stool, fecal enzymes convert urea to ammonia, raising the skin pH and making it more permeable to other irritants. Containment devices, such as external pouches (e.g., rectal, ostomy, perianal), indwelling catheters,[3] incontinence pads and briefs to wick moisture away from the skin, are additional methods to protect patient skin.[6,7]

Steps in a Skin Maintenance Regimen:[3]
1. Cleanse skin with a pH balanced cleanser as soon as it is soiled
   - Cleansing of the skin after each fecal incontinence episode is important because briefs can trap stool against the skin.
2. Moisturize and lubricate skin. Moisturizers may be incorporated into commercially prepared skin cleansers.
3. Apply a skin protectant (sealant, ointment and paste) depending on need:
   - Skin sealants protect the skin from maceration, but have limited effectiveness at protecting the skin from enzymes.
   - Moisture barrier ointments protect the skin from enzymes, but may be inadequate if excessive moisture is present.
   - Pastes are appropriate with high-volume output or diarrhea.

Shear injury:
Occurs when the skin remains stationary and the underlying tissue shifts. Most shear injuries can be eliminated by proper positioning technique. Shear is exerted on the body when the head of the bed is elevated; the skin is fixed against the linens, and the deep fascia and skeleton slide down toward the foot of the bed. Shear also occurs when the individual sitting in a chair slides down in the chair.[8]

Friction injury:
Occurs when the skin moves across a coarse surface, such as bed linens. Voluntary and involuntary movement by patients can lead to friction injuries, especially on elbows and heels. Most friction injuries can be avoided by using proper positioning and transfer techniques. Do not transfer patients by dragging them across the linens. Friction is common in individuals who cannot lift sufficiently during a position change or transfer.[8]

Body Positioning Pressure Points

Body Positions at Risk of Shear and Friction Injury

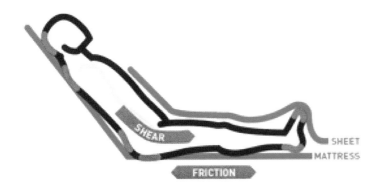

Body Positions at Risk of Pressure Ulcer Formation

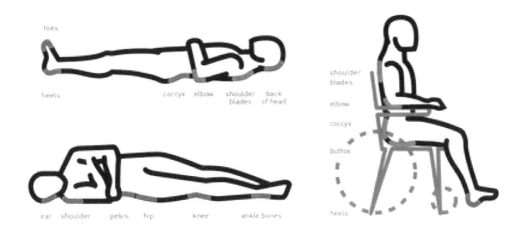

Diagrams ©2012 Aeda Healthcare. Source: http://www.aeda.com

References Chapter 3

1. Alvarez OM, Kalinski C, Nusbaum J, Hernandez L, Pappous E, Kyriannis C, et al. Incorporating wound healing strategies to improve palliation (symptom management) in patients with chronic wounds. *J Palliat Med* 2007;10(5):1161-1189

2. Hess CT. Managing tissue loads. *Adv Skin Wound Care* 2008;21(3):144

3. Bryant RA. Types of skin damage and differential diagnosis. In Bryant RA, Nix DP, eds. *Acute & Chronic Wounds: Current Management Concepts.* 4th ed. St Louis, MO:Elsevier/Mosby. © 2012, p83-107

4. Wound Union of Wound Healing Societies (WUWHS). Woundpedia: evidence informed practice: Ostomy/Continence/Skin Care. [Internet] Available from: http://www.woundpedia.com/ Accessed 6/6/2012

5. Pieper B. Pressure ulcers: impact, etiology, and classification. In Bryant RA, Nix DP, eds. *Acute & Chronic Wounds: Current Management Concepts.* 4th ed. St Louis, MO:Elsevier/Mosby. © 2012, p123-136

6. Ratliff CR. WOCN's evidence-based pressure ulcer guidelines. *Adv Skin Wound Care* 2005;18(4):204-208

7. Institute for Clinical Systems Improvement (ICSI). *Health Care Protocol: Skin safety protocol: risk assessment and prevention of pressure ulcers.* March 2007. [Internet] Available from: http://www.njha.com/qualityinstitute/pdf/226200833420PM63.pdf. Accessed 6/6/2012.

8. Agency for Health Care Policy and Research (AHCPR). *Pressure ulcers in adults: prediction and prevention.* Clinical Practice Guideline no.3; AHCPR-92-0047, May 1992. [Internet] Available from: http://www.eric.ed.gov/PDFS/ED357247.pdf. Accessed 6/6/2012

Physiological Factors

Comprehensive wound care involves assessing existing and potential physiological co-factors that are contributing to delayed wound healing. Some of these co-factors include optimizing nutrition, controlling blood glucose, maximizing blood flow and oxygenation, and ongoing assessment of medications that impact wound healing.

Wound healing process:
The skin is the largest organ in the human body. Any break in skin integrity, regardless of cause (pressure ulcers, burns, neoplasm, trauma), may impact the health of the patient. Wound healing has four phases: hemostasis, inflammation, proliferation, and remodeling.

1. *Hemostasis:* Occurs within first few hours of the body's normal response to tissue injury, initiating the wound-healing cascade. Acute injuries penetrating the epidermis cause bleeding, activating events designed to control blood loss, control bacteria, and seal disrupted vessels ending with formation of a fibrin clot with aggregated platelets and blood cells.[1]

2. *Inflammatory phase:* Lasts 4 to 6 days after the initial injury. Macrophages work to destroy bacteria and cleanse the wound of microscopic debris. Macrophages replace leukocytes, produce cytokines and growth factors, and convert macromolecules into the amino acids and sugars needed in the wound healing process.[2] Edema, induration, and heat may be observed in the periwound skin. Wounds that stall in the inflammatory phase may transform from acute wounds into chronic wounds.[3]

3. *Proliferative phase:* Lasts 2 to 3 weeks in 2 sub-phases. Phase 1 is the generation of granulation tissue, which appears as red, beefy granules of tissue. Granulation begins only after dead tissue is removed from the wound base. Macrophages release fibroblasts, which stimulate collagen production, to create the foundation of the wound base after debris is removed.[3] Collagen provides tensile strength and structure to the healing tissue.[2] When the wound base is filled with granulation tissue, the wound edges are beginning phase 2, epithelialization. Epithelialization starts from the outside edges and progresses towards the center of the wound, with keratinocytes migrating in from wound margins.[3] Formation of a scar completes the proliferative phase, although the body continues to heal the wound after it is closed.[2]

4. *Remodeling phase:* Lasts from 3 weeks to months or even years. During remodeling, cytokines change the wound matrix and strengthen the collagen support structure, which increases the tensile strength of the scar. Tensile strength cannot be fully restored, but may reach 80% of the original strength of the tissue. The wound is vulnerable to re-injury during the remodeling phase.[3] Consequently, reverse staging of pressure ulcers is not appropriate.

The chemistry of the wound base is what allows an acute wound to heal in a reasonable amount of time and prevents it from becoming a chronic wound. Chronic wounds have a more pathologic process that includes:[3]

- prolonged inflammatory phase
- older less viable cells (cellular senescence)
- deficiency of growth factor receptor sites
- no initial bleeding to trigger hemostasis and healing cascade
- higher level of proteases (protein eating enzymes)

Due to these abnormalities, necrotic tissue and slough (yellow, fibrinous tissue) may accumulate in chronic wounds. Tissue necrosis results from inadequate blood supply. The necrotic tissue contains dead cells and debris from dying cells that have not been cleared by normal biological processes in the inflammatory phase. Accumulation of necrotic tissue or slough promotes colonization of bacteria, preventing repair of the wound. The inflammatory response is prolonged and the process of wound contraction and re-epithelialization is prevented.[4]

Nutrition:

Nutrition in the weeks and months prior to death is often challenging. The need for food and fluids decreases as energy demands lessen with decreased activity. As body systems shut down, intake decreases resulting in dehydration and altered metabolism. Protein-calorie malnutrition and dehydration impair skin turgor, leaving tissue susceptible to new breakdown or negatively impacting healing of existing wounds.[5]

Normal healing requires adequate protein, fat, and carbohydrates, as well as vitamins and minerals. Most diets are a combination of these elements so deficiencies of nutrients are uncommon. Loss of protein and fluids from the wound, as well as the increased demands required to support the wound healing process, may increase patient nutrient needs.[6] Oral nutrition is preferred. Suggest patients with wounds choose foods high in protein, such as milk, eggs, cheese, tuna, fish, and meat. Beneficial snacks include pudding, peanut butter and crackers, protein bars, and ice cream. The patient's condition and goals will ultimately determine his/her intake. For nutritionally compromised individuals, a plan of nutritional support or supplementation may be implemented if consistent with the patient/family goals. Before enteral or parental nutrition is used, a critical review of overall goals and wishes of the patient, family, and care team should be considered.[7] Enteral tube feedings or parental nutrition should be considered only if they are in line with the patient's wishes and the treatment of protein-calorie malnutrition will actually increase the possibility of healing.[6,8] Support for the use of enteral nutrition to prevent or heal pressure ulcers is conflicting. In some instances, the use of PEG tubes has actually been shown to increase the risk of pressure ulcers, particularly in nursing home patients with advanced dementia. Tube feeding necessitates the elevation of the head of the bed (HOB) increasing pressure, shear and friction. Use of feeding tubes has not been found to improve survival or prevent aspiration pneumonia. In addition to the lack of evidence in support for ulcer healing and prevention, patients receiving tube feedings may also experience decreased human interaction as utilization of a PEG tube replaces the personal contact received when the patient is fed by another individual.[9]

Food has strong emotional and symbolic implications encompassing nurturing, cultural and religious traditions, and social values. Nutrition and hydration impact wound healing but cannot prevent an individual with co-morbid conditions from dying. Nutritional goals and interventions need to be compatible with the patient's condition and wishes.[10,11] Although some medications may stimulate appetite, they may also hinder wound healing (corticosteroids, such as prednisone or dexamethasone) or cause adverse effects for patients [e.g., DVT risk with megestrol (Megace®); sedation and xerostomia with mirtazapine (Remeron®)].[12] Therefore, non-pharmacological approaches are recommended for the alert patient able to safely tolerate food and drink.[10]

- Small, frequent meals of preferred food/drink
- Relax dietary restrictions (diabetic, sodium, etc) ordered to treat a specific condition
- Offer supplements to patients with protein, vitamin, or mineral deficiencies
- Keep water or other fluids within easy reach, encouraging small, frequent sips
- Offer easy to swallow comfort foods: gelatin, pudding, ice cream, popsicles, soup, etc. Consider adding protein powder to foods, such as pudding, soups, or milkshakes, to increase protein intake and thereby maximizing healing.

While the Agency for Healthcare Research and Quality (AHRQ) pressure ulcer prevention guideline suggests that a serum albumin of less than 3.5 gm/dL predisposes a patient for increased risk of pressure ulcers, one study reveals that current dietary protein intake is a more independent predictor than this lab value.[7] Empirical evidence is lacking that the use of vitamin and mineral supplements, in the absence of deficiency, prevents pressure ulcers. Avoid supplementing patients without protein, vitamin, or mineral deficiencies. Over-the-counter vitamins and minerals are not regulated by the Food & Drug Administration; subsequently, contents and price can vary. Vitamin C and zinc are often recommended for patients with pressure ulcers. Vitamin C is needed for collagen formation and development of tensile strength during wound healing. Supplementation of 500mg of vitamin C twice a day is safe and relatively inexpensive, but there is no evidence to support this practice. In theory, vitamin C is lost when the body is stressed so patients with chronic wounds may be deficient. Vitamin C is water soluble with any excess excreted in the urine. Use caution in patients with history of kidney stones.[13] Zinc has a role in wound-healing, but as with vitamin C, strong evidence for zinc supplementation is lacking. Zinc deficiency is uncommon; but conditions, such as Crohn's disease, short bowel syndrome, alcoholism, chronic liver and chronic renal disease, malignancies, and diabetes, place the patient at higher risk. Large draining wounds may also contribute to zinc loss. Zinc supplement orders should be time-limited with monitoring for side effects: nausea, vomiting, diarrhea, headaches, and cramps.[14] Despite the lack of evidence regarding nutritional assessment and intervention, maintaining optimal nutrition continues to be part of best practice but must be balanced with the individual patient's condition and goals.[7]

Tissue Perfusion & Oxygenation:
Adequate blood flow and oxygenation is necessary for optimal healing and resistance to infection for acute and chronic wounds. All wounds are relatively hypoxic at the center. A main role of oxygen during repair is that of controlling bacteria within the wound site.[15]

Vasoconstrictors cause tissue hypoxia by adversely affecting the microcirculation and leading to poor wound healing.[16] Byproducts of smoking (nicotine, carbon monoxide, hydrogen cyanide) reduce oxygenation, impair the immune response, reduce fibroblast activity, and increase platelet adhesion and thrombus formation. While smoking is associated with significantly higher infection rates, there is no increase in wound infection with use of the nicotine patch.[1]

Several studies document low oxygen levels associated with obesity. Wound healing problems are more likely to occur in patients who are overweight. Individuals who are severely obese often suffer from a number of related health problems that potentially impact healing: type 2 diabetes, hypertension, CAD, sleep apnea, lower extremity ulcers, GERD, and depression. Factors likely to adversely affect perfusion to the wound bed, and therefore oxygen delivery, include hypovolemia, hypotension, factors producing vasoconstriction (cold temperatures, sympathetic stimulation), vascular disease, and edema.[15]

Correcting tissue hypoxia requires more than simply providing supplemental oxygen. Wound oxygenation may remain unchanged even while the patient is breathing additional oxygen.[15] Normal protective physiologic processes shunt blood from the skin to more vital organs. Chronic dehydration may also lead to shunting of the blood to vital organs. Areas of poorly perfused skin are at increased risk of pressure injury and ulcer.[17]

Managing Bacterial Burden:[18]
All pressure ulcers contain a variety of bacteria. Tissue biopsy, not a superficial swab of the wound, is the only method to accurately determine the qualitative and quantitative assessment of any aerobic and anaerobic organisms present. However, tissue biopsy is often not in line with patient/family goals. Empiric treatment of infection may be acceptable based on clinical signs, including odor, exudate, excessive drainage, bleeding, pain, delayed healing, and discoloration of granulation tissue. Increasing pain and wound breakdown are considered sufficient clinical indicators of infected wounds.[7]

The wound bed preparation concept encourages the clinician to examine the whole patient, not just the hole in the patient, treating the cause, as well as patient-centered concerns. Local wound care can be optimized by addressing 3 components: debridement, bacterial balance, and moisture balance.
All chronic wounds contain bacteria. However, whether the wound is in bacterial balance (no tissue damage) or imbalance (critical colonization and infection) is of primary importance to healing. A contaminated or colonized wound has bacteria on the wound surface (contaminated), but the organisms are not associated with tissue damage or delayed healing (colonization). In a wound that is critically colonized (increased bacterial burden), the body's immune response (inflammation) is initiated. If there is bacterial imbalance, the wound may no longer heal at the expected rate. Ideally, in a healable wound, the wound size should decrease 20-40% after four weeks of appropriate treatment and may

heal in 12 weeks. In an infected wound, bacteria have invaded the deeper and surrounding tissues, resulting in an inflammatory response in and around the wound. Bacteria are multiplying and causing tissue damage. Infected wounds are painful and may increase in size with potential new areas of breakdown.

Host resistance is the ability of the host to resist bacterial invasion and damage by mounting an immune response. Systemic and local factors can decrease host resistance. Systemically, an adequate blood supply (blood perfusion to the wound) is needed for wound healing. Systemic challenges to wound healing include uncontrolled edema, vascular insufficiency, poorly controlled diabetes, smoking, poor nutrition, excess alcohol intake, immunodeficiency disease, and drugs that interfere with the immune system (see table, page 15). At the site of the wound, factors that impair healing are the presence of foreign bodies in the wound, untreated deeper infections such as osteomyelitis, and wounds that are very large.

Most bacteria enter the wound bed through environmental contamination, dressings, the patient's body fluids, or the hands of the patient or health care provider. If surface organisms attach to the tissue and multiply, colonization is established but bacterial balance remains. However, if bacteria continue to multiply, critical colonization and infection may develop. The first sign of infection in the wound may be a delay in the healing process. The body's inflammatory reaction to this surface tissue damage causes an increase in exudate. Exudate may be accompanied by a foul odor due to tissue breakdown and gram-negative and anaerobic organisms. Small areas of yellow to brown slough may be present on the wound surface, leading to surface cell death and tissue necrosis. Debridement of necrotic tissue may be considered if circulation is adequate and debridement is consistent with patient goals of care. Granulation tissue, normally pink, may redden and bleed easily, indicating a possible bacterial imbalance. These signs are localized in the superficial wound bed and are potentially treatable with topical agents, including antimicrobial dressings (see table, page 42). Pain, warmth, and swelling surrounding the wound are suggestive of soft tissue cellulitis. Knowing the length of time since the wound developed may assist in anti-microbial treatment. In general, in wounds present less than one month, gram-positive organisms are a factor. Infected wounds present for more than one month, or in the immune compromised patient (including patients with diabetes), are polymicrobial with gram-positive, gram-negative and anaerobic organisms. A change in wound pain has found to be a leading indicator of infection. Additional indicators of wound infection include cellulitis, malodor, delayed healing, wound deterioration or breakdown, and increased volume of exudate.

The mnemonics NERDS and STONES may be helpful in assessment of wound infection:

NERDS = signs of superficial infection when 2-3 of below are present in wound	
N	Non-healing
E	Exudate
R	Red and bleeding surface granulation tissue
D	Debris on surface (yellow or black necrotic tissue)
S	Smell – unpleasant odor from wound (differentiate from absorbent dressings odors)
Treatment: Topical antimicrobials, silver dressings, moist dressings for autolytic debridement.	

STONES = signs of deeper, systemic infection	
S	Size of wound is bigger
T	Temperature of patient is elevated
O	"O's" Probe to exposed bone, or "Os" – Latin root for opening, or "Osteo" – Latin root for bone
N	New areas of breakdown
E	Exudate, erythema, edema
S	Smell

Adapted from Sibbald et al[18]

Best practice for wound care includes implementing the following:
1. Identify the cause and factors that may interfere with healing and address patient-centered concerns.
2. Differentiate the wound's ability to heal: classify as healable, maintenance, or non-healable wound.
3. Focus on use of topical antiseptics for non-healable or maintenance wounds. Active debridement is generally not appropriate.
4. Determine level of bacterial burden (superficially and/or infection in the deep wound bed).
5. Use topical treatment for superficial increased bacterial burden (NERDS). Monitor response to treatment.
6. Use systemic agents for deep infection (STONES). Monitor response to treatment.
7. Reassess the wound at 1 week, 2 weeks, and 4 weeks for signs of improvement. Wound healing is not always the primary goal in hospice. Consider the patient's need for reduced pain, odor, dressing change frequency, and management of exudate.
8. Do not use topical or systemic antibacterial agents longer than 14 days without weighing the benefits and risks of their use.
9. Empower patients through education about wound bed preparation, treatment plans, and prevention. Develop the plan of care in collaboration with the patient. Clinician awareness of individual socioeconomic, cultural, and psychosocial factors for each patient is essential.

Antimicrobial Classifications: Comparison of Antibiotic, Antifungal, and Antiseptic Activity

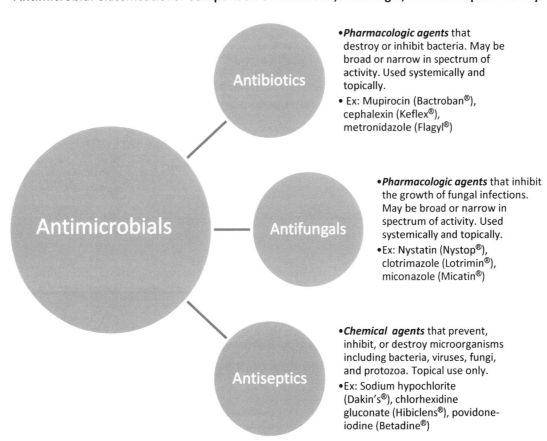

- *Pharmacologic agents* that destroy or inhibit bacteria. May be broad or narrow in spectrum of activity. Used systemically and topically.
- Ex: Mupirocin (Bactroban®), cephalexin (Keflex®), metronidazole (Flagyl®)

- *Pharmacologic agents* that inhibit the growth of fungal infections. May be broad or narrow in spectrum of activity. Used systemically and topically.
- Ex: Nystatin (Nystop®), clotrimazole (Lotrimin®), miconazole (Micatin®)

- *Chemical agents* that prevent, inhibit, or destroy microorganisms including bacteria, viruses, fungi, and protozoa. Topical use only.
- Ex: Sodium hypochlorite (Dakin's®), chlorhexidine gluconate (Hibiclens®), povidone-iodine (Betadine®)

Effects of Medication on Wound Healing[16]

IMPAIR: Medications That May Hinder Wound Healing			
Medication Class	**Examples**	**Mechanism**	**Comments**
Anti-inflammatory	Prednisone, hydrocortisone, dexamethasone, colchicine	Inhibits inflammatory phase of wound healing; impairs granulation and epithelial resurfacing	Corticosteroids help manage other symptoms (pain, appetite, etc); evaluate risk vs. benefits with patient.
Immunosuppressant	Azathioprine, methotrexate, hydroxyurea	May inhibit inflammatory and proliferative phases of wound healing	May no longer be necessary at end of life; evaluate risk vs. benefits with patient.
Antiseptics	Chlorhexidine, povidone iodine, hydrogen peroxide, acetic acid, Dakin's® solution	Change in pH; indiscriminate chemical destruction	Appropriate for cleansing but should not be left on wound bed; rinse with saline after cleansing to minimize toxic effects.
Antibiotics	Mupirocin, gentamicin, bacitracin, neomycin, polymixin B	Topical antibiotics are bacteriostatic only	Topical antibiotics may cause allergic contact dermatitis. Potential for growth of resistant organisms
Cardiovascular -anticoagulants -vasoconstrictors	Warfarin, heparin, epinephrine, nicotine	Prevention of fibrin formation; Vasoconstrictors impair microcirculation	Anticoagulants: Wound healing delayed due to lack of fibrin formation. Vasoconstrictors: decrease blood supply to wound; may increase ulcer necrosis

ENHANCE: Medications That May Benefit Wound Healing			
Medication Class	**Examples**	**Mechanism**	**Comments**
Antiseptics	Chlorhexidine, povidone iodine, acetic acid, Dakin's® solution	Inhibit or destroy microorganisms	Chemical destructive agents to decontaminate wounds. Topical use only. Rinse wound bed with normal saline after use of antiseptics
Anti-epileptics	Phenytoin	Modifies collagen remodeling	May be compounded for topical wound application. See Other Therapies, page 53
Cardiovascular -antiplatelets -vasodilators	Aspirin, NSAIDs, calcium channel blockers	Enhance tissue perfusion through vasodilation or decreased platelet aggregation	Prevents tissue injury through inhibition of thrombus formation. Increases blood flow to ischemic tissue

References Chapter 4

1. Doughty DB, Sparks-DeFriese B. Wound-healing physiology. In Bryant RA, Nix DP, eds. *Acute & Chronic Wounds: Current Management Concepts.* 4th ed. St Louis, MO:Elsevier/Mosby. © 2012, p63-82

2. Hess CT. Understanding the barriers to healing. *Adv Skin Wound Care* 2012;25(5):240

3. Broderick N. Understanding chronic wound healing. *Nurse Practitioner* 2009;34(10):16-22

4. Enoch S, Price P. Cellular, molecular and biochemical differences in the pathophysiology of healing between acute wounds, chronic wounds and wounds in the aged, August 2004. Available at http://www.worldwidewounds.com/2004/august/Enoch/Pathophysiology-Of-Healing.html. Accessed 6/6/2012

5. Langemo D. General principles and approaches to wound prevention and care at the end of life: an overview. *Ostomy Wound Manage* 2012;58(5):24-34

6. Stotts N. Nutritional assessment and support. In Bryant RA, Nix DP, eds. *Acute & Chronic Wounds: Current Management Concepts.* 4th ed. St Louis, MO:Elsevier/Mosby. © 2012, p388-399

7. Lyder CH, Ayello EA. Pressure ulcers: a patient safety issue. In Agency for Healthcare Research and Quality. *Patient Safety and Quality: An Evidence-Based Handbook for Nurses.* AHRQ Pub No. 08-0043, April 2008. [Internet] Available from: http://www.ahrq.gov/qual/nurseshdbk/docs/lyderc_pupsi.pdf. Accessed 6/6/2012

8. Alvarez OM, Kalinski C, Nusbaum J, Hernandez L, Pappous E, Kyriannis C, et al. Incorporating wound healing strategies to improve palliation (symptom management) in patients with chronic wounds. *J Palliat Med* 2007;10(5):1161-1189

9. Teno J, Gozalo P, Mitchell SL, Kuo S, Fulton AT, Mor V. Feeding tubes and the prevention or healing of pressure ulcers. *Arch Intern Med* 2012;172(9):697-701

10. Posthauer ME. Palliative care challenges: offering supportive nutritional care at end of life. [Internet] Available from: http://www.woundsource.com/blog/palliative-care-challenges-offering-supportive-nutritional-care-end-life. Accessed 6/6/2012

11. National Pressure Ulcer Advisory Panel (NPUAP-EPUAP).Pressure Ulcer Prevention and Treatment Guidelines. October 2009

12. Lexi-Comp Online, Lexi-Drugs Online, Hudson, Ohio: Lexi-Comp, Inc.; June 6, 2012

13. Collins N. The facts about vitamin C and wound healing. Ostomy Wound Manage 2009;55(3):8-9

14. Posthauer ME. Does zinc supplementation accelerate wound healing? [Internet] Available from: http://www.woundsource.com/blog/does-zinc-supplementation-accelerate-wound-healing Accessed 11/30/2012

15. Whitney JD. Perfusion and oxygenation. In Bryant RA, Nix DP, eds. *Acute & Chronic Wounds: Current Management Concepts.* 4th ed. St Louis, MO:Elsevier/Mosby. © 2012, p400-407

16. Karukonda SRK, Flynn TC, Boh EE, McBurney EI, Russo GG, Millikan LE. The effects of drugs on wound healing- part II. Specific classes of drugs and their effect on healing wounds. *Int J Dermatol* 2000;39:321-333

17. Sibbald RG, Krasner DL, Lutz J. SCALE: Skin changes at life's end: final consensus statement: October 1, 2009. *Adv Skin Wound Care* 2010;23(5):225-236

18. Sibbald RG, Woo K, Ayello E. Increased bacterial burden and infection: NERDS and STONES. *Adv Skin Wound Care* 2006:19(8):447-461 [Excerpts from this article used with permission from Wulters Kluwer Health, publisher. License no.3083830209509]

Support Surfaces

Pressure-relieving devices are typically the first intervention to prevent development or progression of pressure ulcers.[1] However, support surfaces cannot replace the basic patient care practices of encouraging or assisting with ambulation and repositioning, turning and transferring. These interventions may be scheduled, if necessary, to ensure the routine occurs. If patient ambulation or repositioning is impossible, difficult, or painful, use of the appropriate support surfaces is critical. All support surfaces should meet the following criteria:[2]

- minimize pressure, shear, and friction
- assist in moisture and temperature control
- cleanable surface to minimize contamination
- compatibility with multiple surfaces
- cost effective
- fulfill CMS regulatory requirements
- address patient safety and comfort

The Centers for Medicare and Medicaid Services (CMS) have divided support surfaces into three categories for reimbursement purposes. Only the presence of pressure ulcers determines support surface appropriateness.

Types of Support Surfaces[1,3]

Support Surfaces Category	Description	CMS Guidelines for Use
Group 1	• Static, non-powered • Includes air, foam, gel or water overlays or mattresses	Any patient at risk of developing pressure ulcers
Group 2	• Dynamic, powered • Includes alternating and low-air loss mattresses	Patients who already have partial to full thickness pressure ulcers (stage 2 or worse) May not be CMS reimbursed if used for prevention only
Group 3	• Dynamic, powered • Includes air-fluidized beds only	Patients with non-healing full thickness pressure ulcers (stage 3 or 4) and those who have failed therapy with a Group 2 device

References Chapter 5

1. Alvarez OM, Kalinski C, Nusbaum J, Hernandez L, Pappous E, Kyriannis C, et al. Incorporating wound healing strategies to improve palliation (symptom management) in patients with chronic wounds. *J Palliat Med* 2007;10(5):1161-1189
2. Spahn J. Support surfaces: science and practice. Presented at First Annual Palliative Wound Care Conference, May 13-14, 2010. Hope of Healing Foundation. Cincinnati, Ohio.
3. Lyder CH, Ayello EA. Pressure ulcers: a patient safety issue. In Agency for Healthcare Research and Quality. *Patient Safety and Quality: An Evidence-Based Handbook for Nurses.* AHRQ Pub No. 08-0043, April 2008. [Internet] Available from: http://www.ahrq.gov/qual/nurseshdbk/docs/lyderc_pupsi.pdf. Accessed 6/6/2012

Wound Care Guidance by Type of Wound

Wound care may be guided by the characteristics and type of wound. The following pages contain charts and algorithms to give guidance on wound care based on wound type. Follow the chart through each step or consideration for maintaining the physiologic local wound environment. If debridement is necessary and appropriate, a debridement algorithm provides options for removal of necrotic tissue to aid in wound healing. These steps can also be used to assist in developing and documenting the wound care plan.

These key components are addressed:
- Cleansing
- Debridement
- Dressing selection
- Support surfaces
- Wound symptom management (pain, odor, bleeding, etc)

Note: With any intervention, if improvement is not seen within two weeks consider a change in therapy.

WOUND TREATMENT GRID: Pressure Ulcers Stage 1 & 2

Wound Care Need	Pressure Ulcer Stage 1 or 2	Comments
Description	Stage 1: Localized reddened area, non-blanchable Stage 2: Partial thickness loss of dermis, open/broken blister	Stage 1 may be difficult to detect in patients with darker skin tones
Cleanse	Normal saline or commercial wound cleanser	Irrigate using 4-15 psi: • Spray bottle: 1.2 psi (inadequate) • Piston syringe: 4.2 psi • Squeeze bottle with irrigation cap: 4.5 psi • 35 mL syringe and 18 gauge needle: 8 psi[1] o Proper sharps precautions required if using this method
Debridement	Stage 1 or 2: N/A	No debridement necessary
Dressing	Stage 1: Moisturizer, barrier ointment or cream. Transparent film, thin hydrocolloid, foam. Stage 2: Barrier ointment, Xenaderm® or Granulex®, alginate Transparent film, thin hydrocolloid, foam Contact layer to protect wound bed	• Protect periwound area with a skin barrier film if an adhesive is used • Do not use hydrocolloid if infection is present
Infection	Stage 1: N/A Stage 2:[2] • Honey • Mupirocin (Bactroban®) ointment • Silver dressing • Antiseptics* Use topical antibiotic ≤ 14 days to reduce colonization *Rinse wound bed with normal saline after using any antiseptic cleanser to minimize toxic effects of the antiseptic.*	See Antimicrobials on Wound Care Products chart, page 42. May treat empirically. •MRSA: cadexomer iodine, mupirocin ointment, silver dressing •Pseudomonas: acetic acid 0.25%, topical gentamicin • VRE: hydrofera blue (PVA+methylene blue+gentian violet), silver dressing •MSSA: cadexomer iodine, chlorhexidine, hydrofera blue, mupirocin, silver dressing[2]

Malodor	Stage 1: N/A
	Stage 2:
	• Metronidazole crushed tabs (Flagyl®) to wound bed with dressing changes; use gel (Metrogel®) only if wound bed is dry
	• Charcoal dressings
	• Honey
	• Cleanse with ½ strength (0.25%) sodium hypochlorite (Dakin's® 0.25%)
	• Change hydrocolloid dressing every 24-48 hours.
		• Wound cleansing & debridement aid odor control
		• Change dressing more often to manage odor and/or exudate.
		• Hydrocolloid dressings tend to create odor (doesn't mean infection is present)
		• Environmental strategies:
		  • In room: kitty litter, vanilla extract, coffee grounds, dryer sheets
		  • On dressing: essential oils (wintergreen or lavender)

Dead Space	N/A	N/A
Pruritus	Not usually associated with wound, assess surrounding skin.	If patient reports pruritus, evaluate for contact dermatitis, hypersensitivity, or yeast dermatitis

WOUND TREATMENT GRID: Pressure Ulcers Stage 1 & 2

Wound Care Need	Pressure Ulcer Stage 1 or 2	Comments
Bleeding	Dressing strategies: • Calcium alginate (silver alginate is not hemostatic) • Non-adherent dressing • Coagulants: gelatin sponge, thrombin Topical/local strategies: • Sclerosing agent: silver nitrate • Antifibrinolytic agent: tranexamic acid • Astringents: Alum solution, sucralfate	• Not applicable to Stage 1; skin is intact. • Consider checking: platelet count, PT/INR, vitamin K deficiency • Ask: Is transfusion appropriate? Is patient on warfarin?
Support Surface	Float heels Group 1 Support Surface (prevention) Group 2 Support Surface (stage 2 ulcers present)	• Group 1: Static. Mattress, pressure pad or foam or gel overlays. • Group 2: Dynamic. Alternating and low air loss mattress
Pain	•Topically: - 2% lidocaine or EMLA® cream 30-60 minutes before dressing change;[3] - Morphine in hydrogel (only for open/inflamed wounds)[4] •Systemically: - Pre-medicate 30-60 minutes prior to dressing change with appropriate agent for anxiety and/or for pain. - Neuropathic pain (burning, stabbing, stinging, shooting pain): tricyclic antidepressant, anticonvulsant. - Nociceptive pain: appropriate opioid or corticosteroid	• Allow procedural time-outs. • Use moisture-balanced dressing. • Avoid adherent dressings. • Use warm saline irrigation to remove dressing. • Use contact layer to protect wound bed. • Complementary therapies, such as music, relaxation, aromatherapy, visualization, meditation, can be helpful.

WOUND TREATMENT GRID: Pressure Ulcers Stage 3 & 4

Wound Care Need	Pressure Ulcer Stage 3 or 4	Comments
Description	Stage 3: Full thickness ulcer with subcutaneous tissue visible Stage 4: Full thickness ulcer with exposed muscle, tendon, and/or bone	Stage 3 and 4 ulcers have highest infection risk Osteomyelitis risk if bone is exposed
Cleanse	Normal saline, commercial wound cleanser, *antiseptics: acetic acid 0.25%, chlorhexidine, hydrogen peroxide, povidone-iodine (Betadine®), ½ strength sodium hypochlorite (Dakin's solution 0.25%)	Irrigate with 4-15 psi to remove debris. • Spray bottle: 1.2 psi (inadequate) • Piston syringe: 4.2 psi • Squeeze bottle with irrigation cap: 4.5 psi • 35 mL syringe and 18 gauge needle: 8 psi[1] o Proper sharps precautions required if using this method *Rinse wound bed with normal saline after using any antiseptic cleanser to avoid toxic effects.
Debridement	•Autolytic: transparent dressing, hydrocolloid, alginate; hydrogel if wound is dry. •Chemical: collagenase (Santyl®) (change 1-2 times per day); Full-strength sodium hypochlorite (Dakin's® solution, 0.5%)[5] applied to gauze and packed in wound • Biosurgical: Larval therapy[5]	• See Debridement Algorithm • Silver inactivates collagenase; do not use silver dressing and collagenase together. • Only leave full-strength Dakin's® solution in contact with wound bed if intent is debridement.
Dressing	Hydrocolloid (do not use if infection is present), alginate, foam Contact layer to protect wound bed.	• Protect periwound area with a skin barrier film if an adhesive is used
Infection	• Silver dressing • Honey • Antiseptics[2] • Cleanse with ½ strength sodium hypochlorite (Dakin's® solution 0.25%), then rinse with normal saline • Use topical antibiotics ≤ 14 days to reduce colonization	See Antimicrobials on Wound Care Products chart, page 42. May treat empirically. •MRSA: cadexomer iodine, silver dressing •Pseudomonas: acetic acid • VRE: hydrofera blue, silver dressing • MSSA: cadexomer iodine, chlorhexidine, hydrofera blue, silver dressing *Rinse wound bed with normal saline after using any antiseptic cleanser to minimize toxic effects

Malodor	• Metronidazole crushed tabs (Flagyl®) to wound bed with dressing changes; use gel (Metrogel®) only if wound bed is dry
	• Charcoal dressing
	• Honey
	• Cleanse with ½ strength Dakin's® solution, then rinse with normal saline
	• Change hydrocolloid dressing every 24-48 hours.
		• Wound cleansing & debridement aid in odor control
		• Change dressing more often to manage odor and/or exudate
		• Hydrocolloid dressings tend to create odor (doesn't mean infection is present)
		• Do not use hydrocolloid if infection is present
		• Environmental strategies:
		   • In room: kitty litter, vanilla extract, coffee grounds, dryer sheets
		   • On dressing: essential oils (wintergreen or lavender)

Dead Space	Alginate roping; foam; wound fillers; collagen; hydrogel	Dressing materials placed into open wounds to eliminate dead space, absorb exudate, or maintain moisture
Pruritus	Not usually associated with wound, assess surrounding skin.	If patient reports pruritus, evaluate for contact dermatitis, hypersensitivity, or yeast dermatitis

21

WOUND TREATMENT GRID: Pressure Ulcers Stage 3 & 4

Wound Care Need	Pressure Ulcer Stage 3 or 4	Comments
Bleeding	Dressing strategies: • Calcium alginate (silver alginate is not hemostatic) • Non-adherent dressing • Coagulants: gelatin sponge, thrombin Topical/local strategies: • Sclerosing agent: silver nitrate • Antifibrinolytic agent: tranexamic acid • Astringents: Alum solution, sucralfate • Vasoconstrictive agents: topical oxymetazoline (Afrin®) , topical epinephrine	• Consider checking: platelet count, PT/INR, vitamin K deficiency. • Ask: Is transfusion appropriate? Is patient on warfarin? • Use topical vasoconstrictors only when bleeding is minimal, oozing, or seeping
Support Surface	Group 2 Support Surface: Any patient with partial to full thickness ulcers already present. Group 3 Support Surface: Patient must have large or multiple stage 3 or 4 pressure ulcers on trunk or pelvis, be bedbound, and all alternative measures have failed (criteria to receive Medicare reimbursement).	•Group 2: Dynamic. Powered air flotation beds & pressure reducing air mattress, non-powered advanced pressure reducing mattress •Group 3: Dynamic. Air-fluidized bed
Pain	•Topically: - 2% lidocaine or EMLA® cream 30-60 minutes before dressing change;[3] - Morphine in hydrogel (only for open/inflamed wounds)[4] •Systemically: - Pre-medicate 30-60 minutes prior to dressing change with appropriate agent for anxiety and/or for pain. - Neuropathic pain (burning, stabbing, stinging, shooting pain): tricyclic antidepressant, anticonvulsant. - Nociceptive pain: appropriate opioid or corticosteroid	• Allow procedural time-outs. • Use moisture-balanced dressing. • Use appropriate irrigation force. • Avoid adherent dressings. • Use warm saline irrigation to remove dressing. • Use contact layer to protect wound bed. • Complementary therapies, such as music, relaxation, aromatherapy, visualization, meditation, can be helpful.

DEBRIDEMENT ALGORITHM: Pressure Ulcers Stage 3 or 4

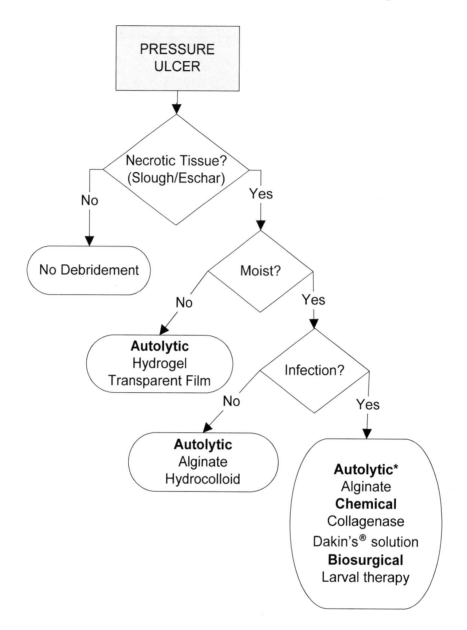

Use in conjunction with the appropriate topical antimicrobial

- See Wound Treatment Grid for additional symptom management
- See Types of Debridement Chart for more information

WOUND TREATMENT GRID: Stable Eschar

Wound Care Need	Stable Eschar	Comments
Description	Thick, leathery, black or brown crust; nonviable tissue, colonized with bacteria	Stable eschar is defined as firmly adherent, hard, non-infected and dry
Cleanse	Paint with antiseptic solution, e.g. povidone-iodine (Betadine®)[6]	Leave open to air
Debridement	Do not debride stable eschar (non-infected, dry)[5]	See Debridement Algorithm
Dressing	If on heel, paint with povidone-iodine (Betadine®) and leave open to air[7]	
Infection	Not considered stable if signs of infection present	
Malodor	If there's odor, it's probably not stable.	
Dead Space	N/A	Cannot be determined if eschar is present.
Pruritus	Not usually associated with wound, assess surrounding skin.	If patient reports pruritus, evaluate for contact dermatitis, hypersensitivity, or yeast dermatitis
Bleeding	Not considered stable if bleeding is present	
Support Surface	Varies by wound location. If on heel: elevate calves on longitudinal pillows, thereby "floating the heels"; static heel boots or foam boots--*not* "Moon Boots"	•Group 1: Static. Mattress, pressure pad or overlay •Group 2: Dynamic. Powered air flotation beds & pressure reducing air mattress, non-powered advanced pressure reducing mattress •Group 3: Dynamic. Air-fluidized bed
Pain	Medicate with appropriate agent for anxiety and/or for pain. • Neuropathic pain (burning, stabbing, stinging, shooting pain): tricyclic antidepressant, anticonvulsant • Nociceptive pain (gnawing, throbbing, tenderness): opioid or corticosteroid	

DEBRIDEMENT ALGORITHM: Eschar

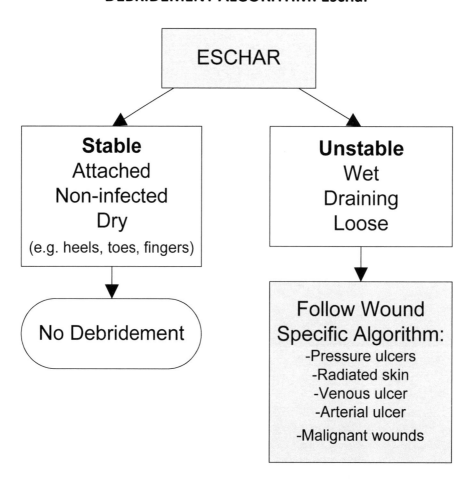

ESCHAR

Stable
Attached
Non-infected
Dry

(e.g. heels, toes, fingers)

No Debridement

Unstable
Wet
Draining
Loose

Follow Wound
Specific Algorithm:
-Pressure ulcers
-Radiated skin
-Venous ulcer
-Arterial ulcer
-Malignant wounds

- See Wound Treatment Grid for additional symptom management
- See Types of Debridement Chart for more information

WOUND TREATMENT GRID: Arterial or Ischemic Ulcers

Wound Care Need	Arterial Ulcer/Ischemic Ulcer	Comments
Description	Shallow well-defined borders, pale wound bed	Usually on tips of toes or between toes but may also be on lateral malleolus
Cleanse	Normal saline or commercial wound cleanser If stable eschar is present, paint with povidone-iodine (Betadine®).	Irrigate with 4-15 psi: • Spray bottle: 1.2 psi (inadequate) • Piston syringe: 4.2 psi • Squeeze bottle with irrigation cap: 4.5 psi • 35 mL syringe and 18 gauge needle: 8 psi[1] o Proper sharps precautions required if using this method
Debridement	Debridement not recommended unless perfusion status is determined, i.e. toe pressures and transcutaneous oxygen measurements •**Autolytic**: Hydrogel, alginate, hydrocolloid.[8] If dry, intact, non-infected eschar do not remove[6]	• See Debridement Algorithm
Dressing	• Hydrogel • Hydrocolloid (do not use if infection is present) • Foam • If stable eschar is present, leave open to air.	• Protect periwound area with a skin barrier film if an adhesive is used • Usually minimal exudate
Infection	• Silver impregnated dressing • Consider systemic antibiotic therapy[6] • Use topical antibiotics ≤ 14 days to reduce colonization risk	See Antimicrobials on Wound Care Products chart, page 42. May treat empirically. •MRSA: cadexomer iodine, mupirocin ointment, silver dressing •Pseudomonas: acetic acid • VRE: hydrofera blue, silver dressing • MSSA: cadexomer iodine, chlorhexidine, hydrofera blue, mupirocin, silver dressing

Malodor	• Metronidazole crushed tabs (Flagyl®) to wound bed with dressing changes; use gel (Metrogel®) only if wound bed is dry
	• Charcoal dressing
	• Honey
	• Change hydrocolloid dressing every 24-48 hours.
		• Wound cleansing aids odor control
		• Change dressing more often to manage odor and/or exudate
		• Hydrocolloid dressings tend to create odor (doesn't mean infection is present)
		• Environmental strategies:
		  • In room: kitty litter, vanilla extract, coffee grounds, dryer sheets
		  • On dressing: essential oils (wintergreen or lavender)

Dead Space	Alginate roping, pastes or powders, collagen	Dressing materials placed into open wounds to eliminate dead space, absorb exudate, or maintain moisture.
Pruritus	Not usually associated with wound, assess surrounding skin.	If patient reports pruritus, evaluate for contact dermatitis, hypersensitivity, or yeast dermatitis

WOUND TREATMENT GRID: Arterial or Ischemic Ulcers

Wound Care Need	Arterial Ulcer/Ischemic Ulcer	Comments
Bleeding	Dressing strategies: • Calcium alginate (silver alginate is not hemostatic) • Non-adherent dressing • Coagulants: gelatin sponge, thrombin Topical/local strategies: • Sclerosing agent: silver nitrate • Antifibrinolytic agent: tranexamic acid • Astringents: Alum solution, sucralfate	• Consider checking: platelet count, PT/INR, vitamin K deficiency. • Ask: Is transfusion appropriate? Is patient on warfarin?
Support Surface	N/A. Only *pressure ulcers* determine use of support surfaces	• Medicare reimbursement is based on presence of *pressure ulcers*, not other wound types.
Pain	• Pain is often severe-even at rest • Elevation of extremity may increase pain; dangling legs over side of bed may relieve pain • Consider antiplatelet agents: cilostazol (Pletal®) • Pre-medicate with appropriate agent for pain and/or anxiety prior to dressing change • Neuropathic pain (burning, stabbing, stinging, shooting pain): tricyclic antidepressant, anticonvulsant • Nociceptive pain (gnawing, throbbing, tenderness): opioid or corticosteroid	• Allow procedural time-outs. • Use moisture-balanced dressing. • Avoid adherent dressings. • Use warm saline irrigation to remove dressing. • Complementary therapies, such as music, relaxation, aromatherapy, visualization, meditation, can be helpful. • Cilostazol (Pletal®) is contraindicated in patients with heart failure - any level of severity.
Other	• Characteristics: minimal exudate; infection common, including gangrene, • Pulses may or may not be present • Thin, fragile skin[9] • Ulcer is due to occlusion of one or more arteries • Use lamb's wool or foam toe sleeves to prevent interdigital friction	• Do not use hot water bottles, heating pads or other thermal devices. • These ulcers are also known as LEAD-Lower Extremity Arterial Ulcers. • Calciphylaxis associated with end stage renal disease (ESRD) see Special Topics, page 47.

DEBRIDEMENT ALGORITHM: Arterial Ulcer

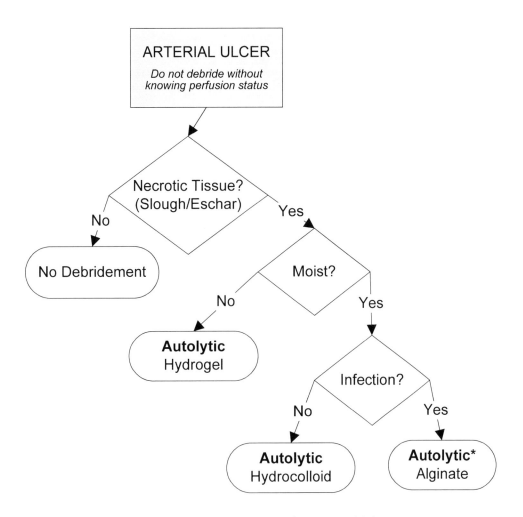

Use in conjunction with the appropriate topical antimicrobial

- See Wound Treatment Grid for additional symptom management
- See Types of Debridement Chart for more information

WOUND TREATMENT GRID: Venous Ulcers

Wound Care Need	Venous Ulcer	Comments
Description	• Usually shallow with irregular edges; often heavy exudate • 70-90% of leg ulcers are venous ulcers	Characteristics: • Usually lower legs between ankles and knees • Ruddy skin; edema; pulses usually present
Cleanse	Normal saline or commercial wound cleanser	Irrigate with 4-15 psi: • Spray bottle: 1.2 psi (inadequate) • Piston syringe: 4.2 psi • Squeeze bottle with irrigation cap: 4.5 psi • 35 mL syringe and 18 gauge needle: 8 psi[1] ○ Proper sharps precautions required if using this method
Debridement	• Autolytic: alginate if wound is moist; hydrogel if wound is dry • Sharp debridement • Enzymatic debridement[8]: collagenase (Santyl®)	See Debridement Algorithm Consider checking an ankle brachial index (ABI) for chronic, non-healing leg ulcers. Silver inactivates collagenase; therefore, do not use silver and collagenase together.
Dressing	• Foam, alginate[8], hydrogel • Contact layer to protect wound bed	• Protect periwound area with skin barrier film if an adhesive is used, otherwise protect periwound area from maceration with barrier cream or ointment. • All lower extremity wounds should be bandaged due to heavy exudate, to minimize infection • Usually moderate to heavy exudate
Infection	• Topical: silver dressing, antiseptics • Use topical antibiotics ≤ 14 days to reduce colonization risk • Systemic antibiotics	See Antimicrobials on Wound Care Products chart, page 42. May treat empirically. •MRSA: cadexomer iodine, mupirocin ointment, silver dressing •Pseudomonas: acetic acid 0.25% • VRE: hydrofera blue, silver dressing • MSSA: cadexomer iodine, chlorhexidine, hydrofera blue, mupirocin silver dressing[10]

Malodor	• Metronidazole crushed tabs (Flagyl®) to wound bed with dressing changes; use gel (Metrogel®) only if wound bed is dry
	• Charcoal dressing
	• Honey
	• Increase frequency of dressing change
		• Wound cleansing aids odor control.
		• Change dressing more often to manage odor and/or exudate.
		• Hydrocolloid dressings tend to create odor (doesn't mean infection is present)
		• Environmental strategies:
		  • In room: kitty litter, vanilla extract, coffee grounds, dryer sheets
		  • On dressing: essential oils (wintergreen or lavender)

Dead Space	Alginate roping, pastes or powders, collagen	

WOUND TREATMENT GRID: Venous Ulcers

Wound Care Need	Venous Ulcer	Comments
Pruritus	Topical: • Apply unscented, lanolin free hydrophilic moisturizers: Lubriderm®, Eucerin®, Keri®, Aquaphor®[11] • Corticosteroid creams (start with OTC first): Cortaid®, Kenalog®	• Due to skin changes with chronic venous insufficiency, dermatitis and pruritus are common. • Skin changes may mimic cellulitis. Avoid antibiotics unless known bacterial infection is present. • Stasis dermatitis usually responds to moisturizer • Corticosteroids may be needed to reduce pruritus, usually topical. May use burst of oral corticosteroids if severe.
Bleeding	Dressing strategies: • Calcium alginate (silver alginate is not hemostatic) • Non-adherent dressing • Coagulants: gelatin sponge, thrombin Topical/local strategies: • Sclerosing agent: silver nitrate • Antifibrinolytic agent: tranexamic acid • Astringents: Alum solution, sucralfate	• Consider checking: platelet count, PT/INR, vitamin K deficiency • Ask: Is transfusion appropriate? Is patient on warfarin?
Support Surface	N/A. Only *pressure ulcers* determine use of support surfaces	Medicare reimbursement is based on presence of *pressure ulcers*, not other wound types.
Pain	• Usually a dull aching pain or heaviness that is relieved as edema decreases • Elevation of the extremity may decrease pain even without presence of edema • Pre-medicate with appropriate agent for pain and/or anxiety prior to dressing change • Neuropathic pain (burning, stabbing, stinging, shooting pain): tricyclic antidepressant, anticonvulsant • Nociceptive pain (gnawing, throbbing, tenderness): opioid or corticosteroid	• Allow procedural time-outs. • Use moisture-balanced dressing. • Use appropriate irrigation force. • Avoid adherent dressings. • Use warm saline irrigation to remove dressing. • Complementary therapies, such as music, relaxation, aromatherapy, visualization, meditation, can be helpful.
Other	• Shallow wound base with granulation tissue-rarely necrotic • Edema is one of the early signs • Hyperpigmentation of calves	Compression therapy is usually part of venous ulcer management. For additional information see Special Topics, page 52.

DEBRIDEMENT ALGORITHM: Venous Ulcer

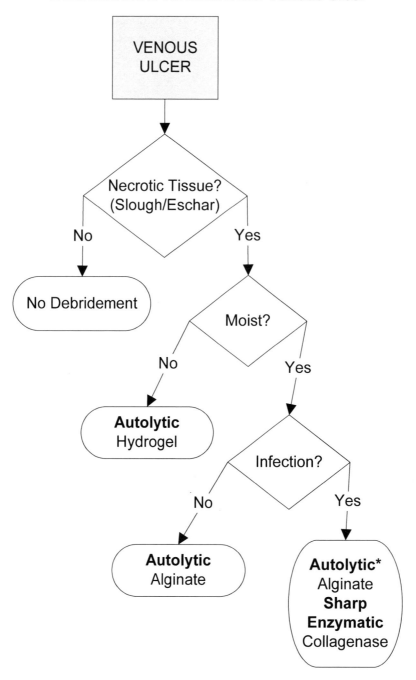

Use in conjunction with the appropriate topical antimicrobial

- See Wound Treatment Grid for additional symptom management
- See Types of Debridement Chart for more information

WOUND TREATMENT GRID: Radiated Skin

Wound Care Need	Radiated Skin	Comments
Description	• Damaged by radiation therapy; appears burned, crusty, peeling, or friable • Usually fairly superficial, but is possible for the wound to be deeper	• Any radiated area of body • May include hair loss to the area, decreased perspiration, superficial changes to blood vessels, edema, and scarring[12] • Inflammation usually occurs immediately after area is radiated
Cleanse	Use lukewarm water & mild non-alkaline soap: baby soap, Dove®, or Ivory®[11]	• Hydrogel for desquamation (removal of scaling) • Normal saline soaks to loosen crusting • Do not rub skin-pat dry
Debridement	Don't usually debride	• See Debridement Algorithm • Consult physician re: surgical debridement if appropriate
Topical Treatment	• Apply unscented, lanolin-free hydrophilic moisturizers: Lubriderm®, Eucerin®, Keri®, Aquaphor®[11] • Corticosteroid cream for erythema • Hydrogel: dry desquamation • Foam: moist desquamation	• Protect periwound area with a skin barrier film if an adhesive is used • Cover wound to minimize evaporation, pain, and risk of infection • Apply moisturizer 2-3 times/day • Protect from sun with SPF 15 or higher • Protect from friction, rubbing, or tight clothes • Protect from extreme heat/cold, cuts, and scrapes
Infection	• Topical antibiotics helpful as this damaged tissue is less able to resist or fight infection[12] • Use topical antibiotics ≤ 14 days to reduce colonization risk	See Antimicrobials on Wound Care Products chart, page 42. May treat empirically. •MRSA: cadexomer iodine, mupirocin ointment, silver dressing •Pseudomonas: acetic acid 0.25% • VRE: hydrofera blue, silver dressing • MSSA: cadexomer iodine, chlorhexidine, hydrofera blue, mupirocin silver dressing[10]
Malodor	• Honey • Topical metronidazole (Flagyl®)	
Dead Space	N/A	
Pruritus	• Topical corticosteroid creams • Normal saline compresses • Cool mist humidifier • Cooled hydrogel sheets	If patient reports pruritus, evaluate for contact dermatitis, hypersensitivity, or yeast dermatitis
Bleeding	Not likely, but may occur	Encourage gentle cleansing and moisturizers
Support Surface	N/A. Only *pressure ulcers* determine use of support surfaces	Medicare reimbursement is based on presence of *pressure ulcers*, not other wound types.
Pain	• Aloe vera gel may soothe and cool radiated skin • Morphine in hydrogel (only for open/inflamed wounds)[4]	• Allow procedural time-outs. • Use moisture-balanced, dressing. • Use appropriate irrigation force. • Avoid adherent dressings or clothing. • Complementary therapies, such as music, relaxation, aromatherapy, visualization, meditation, can be helpful.
Other	Do not use petrolatum based products, products with perfumes or alpha-hydroxy acids[11]	

DEBRIDEMENT ALGORITHM: Radiated Skin

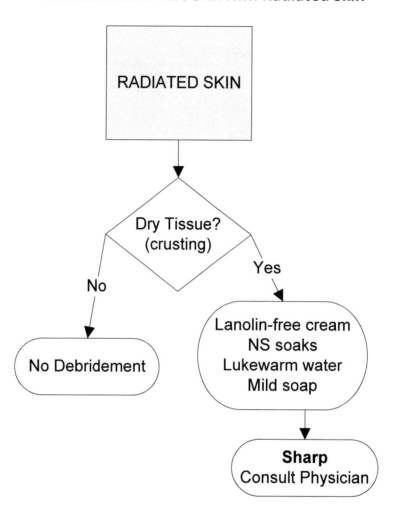

- See Wound Treatment Grid for additional symptom management
- See Types of Debridement Chart for more information

WOUND TREATMENT GRID: Fungating/Malignant Wounds

Wound Care Need	Fungating/Malignant	Comments
Description	May be primary cutaneous tumor, metastatic disease, or malignant transformation of wound[13]	<ul><li>Exudate, odor, and bleeding often contribute to psychosocial issues.</li><li>Healing is rare</li><li>Marjolin ulcer: malignant transformation of a chronic wound, occurs in 2% of chronic wounds[13]</li></ul>
Cleanse	<ul><li>Normal saline or commercial wound cleanser</li><li>Irrigate instead of swabbing to minimize bleeding</li></ul>	Irrigate with 4-15 psi:<ul><li>Spray bottle: 1.2 psi (inadequate)</li><li>Piston syringe: 4.2 psi</li><li>Squeeze bottle with irrigation cap: 4.5 psi</li><li>35 mL syringe and 18 gauge needle: 8 psi[1]<ul><li>Proper sharps precautions required if using this method</li></ul></li></ul>
Debridement	<ul><li>Autolytic: transparent dressing, alginate; hydrogel if wound is dry.</li><li>Enzymatic: collagenase (Santyl®)</li></ul>	See Debridement Algorithm
Dressing	<ul><li>Foam, alginate, hydrofiber based on wound need</li><li>Moisture is usually contraindicated</li><li>Avoid hydrating gels & hydrocolloids[14]</li></ul>	<ul><li>Protect periwound area with a skin barrier film if an adhesive is used</li></ul>
Infection	Topical:<ul><li>Mupirocin ointment</li><li>Silver dressing</li><li>Antiseptics*</li></ul>Use topical antibiotics ≤ 14 days to reduce colonization risk	See Antimicrobials on Wound Care Products chart, page 42. May treat empirically. •MRSA: cadexomer iodine, mupirocin ointment, silver dressing •Pseudomonas: acetic acid 0.25%, topical gentamicin • VRE: hydrofera blue, silver dressing •MSSA: cadexomer iodine, chlorhexidine, hydrofera blue, mupirocin, silver dressing *Rinse wound bed with normal saline after using any antiseptic cleanser to minimize toxic effects.
Malodor	<ul><li>Metronidazole crushed tabs (Flagyl®) to wound bed with dressing changes; use gel (Metrogel®) only if wound bed is dry</li><li>Charcoal dressings</li><li>Honey</li><li>Increase frequency of dressing change</li></ul>	<ul><li>Wound cleansing & debridement aid odor control.</li><li>Change dressing more often to manage odor and/or exudate.</li><li>Environmental strategies:<ul><li>In room: kitty litter, vanilla extract, coffee grounds, dryer sheets</li><li>On dressing: essential oils (wintergreen or lavender)</li></ul></li></ul>
Dead Space	N/A	
Pruritus	Not usually associated with wound, assess surrounding skin.	If patient reports pruritus, evaluate for contact dermatitis, hypersensitivity, or yeast dermatitis

WOUND TREATMENT GRID: Fungating/Malignant Wounds

Wound Care Need	Fungating/Malignant	Comments
Bleeding	Radiation therapy (short course) may be appropriate for bleeding tumors of the breast or skin Dressing strategies: • Calcium alginate (silver alginate is not hemostatic) • Non-adherent dressing • Coagulants: gelatin sponge, thrombin • Acute event dressings: Quikclot®, Celox® Topical/local strategies: • Sclerosing agent: silver nitrate • Antifibrinolytic agent: tranexamic acid • Astringents: Alum solution, sucralfate • Epinephrine (1:1000) spray • Topical thrombin • Oxymetalozine (Afrin®) spray Oral: Tranexamic acid	• Tissue is friable and predisposed to bleeding • Prepare patient/caregivers for possible hemorrhage (dark towels & bed linens) • Consider checking: platelet count, PT/INR, vitamin K deficiency • Ask: Is transfusion appropriate? Is patient on warfarin?
Support Surface	N/A. Only *pressure ulcers* determine use of support surfaces	Medicare reimbursement is based on presence of *pressure ulcers*, not other wound types.
Pain	Topical: • 2% lidocaine or EMLA® cream 30-60 min before dressing change[3] • Ketamine (see *Other Therapies*, p53) • Morphine in hydrogel (only for open/inflamed wounds)[4] Systemic: • Pre-medicate with appropriate agent for pain and/or anxiety prior to dressing change • Neuropathic pain (burning, stabbing, stinging, shooting pain): tricyclic antidepressant, anticonvulsant • Nociceptive pain (gnawing, throbbing, tenderness): opioid or corticosteroid	• Allow procedural time-outs. • Use moisture-balanced dressing. • Use appropriate irrigation force. • Avoid adherent dressings. • Use warm saline irrigation to remove dressing. • Contact layer protects wound bed. • Complementary therapies, such as music, relaxation, aromatherapy, visualization, meditation, can be helpful.

DEBRIDEMENT ALGORITHM: Fungating/Malignant Wounds

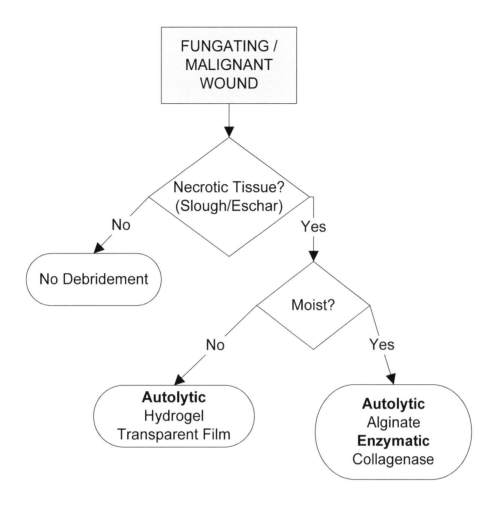

FUNGATING /
MALIGNANT
WOUND

Necrotic Tissue?
(Slough/Eschar)

No

No Debridement

Yes

Moist?

No

Autolytic
Hydrogel
Transparent Film

Yes

Autolytic
Alginate
Enzymatic
Collagenase

- See Wound Treatment Grid for additional symptom management
- See Types of Debridement Chart for more information

References Chapter 6

1. Sibbald RG, Krasner DL, Lutz J. SCALE: Skin changes at life's end: final consensus statement: October 1, 2009. *Adv Skin Wound Care* 2010;23(5):225-236

2. Rolstad BS, Bryant RA, Nix DP. Topical management. In Bryant RA, Nix DP, eds. *Acute & Chronic Wounds: Current Management Concepts.* 4th ed. St Louis, MO:Elsevier/Mosby. © 2012, p289-306

3. Hopf HW, Shapshak D, Junkins S. Managing wound pain. In Bryant RA, Nix DP, eds. *Acute & Chronic Wounds: Current Management Concepts.* 4th ed. St Louis, MO:Elsevier/Mosby. © 2012, p380-387

4. Tran QNH, Fancher T. Achieving analgesia for painful ulcers using topically applied morphine gel. J Support Oncol 2007;5(6):289-293

5. Ramundo J. Wound debridement. In Bryant RA, Nix DP, eds. *Acute & Chronic Wounds: Current Management Concepts.* 4th ed. St Louis, MO:Elsevier/Mosby. © 2012, p279-288

6. Doughty DB. Arterial ulcers. In Bryant RA, Nix DP, eds. *Acute & Chronic Wounds: Current Management Concepts.* 4th ed. St Louis, MO:Elsevier/Mosby. © 2012, p178-193

7. American Association for Long Term Care Nursing (AALTCN). Ask the Wound Coach. [Internet] Available from: http://ltcnursing.org/ask-the-wound-coach.htm. Accessed 6/6/2012

8. Lippincott, Williams and Wilkins. Wound Care Made Incredibly Visual. 2nd Edition.

9. Ermer-Selton J. Lower extremity assessment. In Bryant RA, Nix DP, eds. *Acute & Chronic Wounds: Current Management Concepts.* 4th ed. St Louis, MO:Elsevier/Mosby. © 2012, p169-177

10. Stotts N. Wound infection: diagnosis and management. In Bryant RA, Nix DP, eds. *Acute & Chronic Wounds: Current Management Concepts.* 4th ed. St Louis, MO:Elsevier/Mosby. © 2012, p270-278

11. Bryant RA. Types of skin damage and differential diagnosis. In Bryant RA, Nix DP, eds. *Acute & Chronic Wounds: Current Management Concepts.* 4th ed. St Louis, MO:Elsevier/Mosby. © 2012, p83-107

12. Langemo D. General principles and approaches to wound prevention and care at the end of life: an overview. *Ostomy Wound Manage* 2012;58(5):24-34

13. Goldberg MT, Bryant RA. Managing wounds in palliative care. In Bryant RA, Nix DP, eds. *Acute & Chronic Wounds: Current Management Concepts.* 4th ed. St Louis, MO:Elsevier/Mosby. © 2012, p505-513

14. Woo KY, Sibbald RG. Local wound care for malignant and palliative wounds. Adv Skin Wound Care. 2010;23(9):417-428

15. Patel B, Cox-Hayley D. Managing wound odor. *Fast Facts & Concepts.* August 2009; 218. Available at http://www.eperc.mcw.edu/EPERC/FastFactsIndex/ff_218.htm. Accessed 6/6/2012

Product Selection by Wound Condition

Using Wound Condition to Assist in Product Selection

CONDITION	PRODUCT & DESCRIPTION	INDICATION	COMMENTS
PERIWOUND PROTECTION	**Skin Barrier Film:** • Liquid transparent film that contains plasticizing agents • Available as a spray or wipe • Some contain isopropyl alcohol *Brands: No Sting Skin Prep, Cavilon No Sting Barrier*	• Use around wound, before applying dressing, to protect surrounding skin from maceration, skin stripping and infection.	• Use non-alcohol based product if surrounding skin is compromised • Also known as "skin sealant" • Alcohol free products: Cavilon No Sting®, No Sting Skin Prep®

WOUND CLEANSING	**Wound Cleanser:**
	• Cleanser of choice: Normal saline
	• If no preservative, replace every 24 hours
	• Commercial products: follow product specific expiration dating
	Brands: ALLCLENZ, Cavilon, DermaKlenz, Skintegrity, normal saline
		• Gentle irrigation preferred over swabbing
		• If suspect colonization/infection, irrigate with antiseptic or antimicrobial agent
		• Rinse with normal saline after cleansing with antiseptic.
		• Irrigation removes surface bacteria & debris
			• Every wound requires cleansing with each dressing change to remove surface bacteria and debris.[24]
			• Surfactants in commercial wound cleanser help lift debris from the wound bed
			• Irrigation force 4-15 psi:
			  • Spray bottle: 1.2 psi (inadequate)
			  • Piston syringe: 4.2 psi
			  • Squeeze bottle with irrigation cap: 4.5 psi
			  • 35 mL syringe and 18 gauge needle: 8 psi
			  (Proper sharps precautions required if using this method)

	Transparent Film: • Occlusive, transparent, adhesive, non-absorbent • Permeable to oxygen and water vapor; impermeable to bacteria and contaminants *Brands: Opsite, Suresite, Tegaderm*	• Dry to minimal exudate • Shallow or partial thickness wounds • Supports autolytic debridement • Maintains moist wound surface • Used as a cover dressing • Provides protection from friction, shear, microbes, & chemicals • Allows visualization of wound	• Not for exudative wounds • Not for infected wounds • Does not adhere well in moist areas • Need 2 inch border around wound • Change every 3-7 days or if exudate is beyond wound border.
DRY WOUND BED	**Hydrogel:** • Water or glycerin-based amorphous gel, sheet or impregnated gauze that hydrates *Brands: Skintegrity, Vigilon*	• Dry to minimal exudate • Partial or full-thickness wounds without depth • Supports autolytic debridement • Softens necrotic tissue • Donates moisture • Decreases pain	• Not for heavily draining wounds • Change sheet form every 1-3 days. • Change sterile gel form every 3 days; change non-sterile gel every day • Sheets without borders require secondary dressing • Apply skin barrier ointment or skin sealant to immediate periwound skin to prevent maceration.

Using Wound Condition to Assist in Product Selection

CONDITION	PRODUCT & DESCRIPTION	INDICATION	COMMENTS
MINIMAL TO MODERATE EXUDATE	**Hydrocolloid:** • Occlusive wafer dressing • Forms gelatinous mass to reduce wound contamination • Water resistant outer layer *Brands: Duoderm, Exuderm, Replicare, Tegasorb*	• Minimal to moderate exudative wound with slough present • Partial or full thickness wounds without depth • Supports autolytic debridement • Maintains moist wound surface • Provides pain relief	• Not for infected wounds or wounds with deep tunnels, tracts & undermining • Not for wounds with stable eschar • Occlusive properties can promote infection in high risk patients • Change every 3-5 days or when fluid leaks from under wafer • Dislodges with heavy exudate, shearing or friction • May tear fragile surrounding skin –use periwound skin sealant • Can develop foul odor after 2-4 days –may be mistaken for infection
	Alginate: • Derived from brown seaweed • Forms moisture retentive gel on contact with wound fluid • Rope or flat dressing forms • Calcium alginate is hemostatic • Silver alginate is antimicrobial • Holds up to 20x its weight in fluid • Layer for increased absorption *Brands: Algiderm, Algisite, Algicel, Kaltostat, Restore CalciCare, Sorbsan, Tegagen*	• Moderate to heavy exudate • Partial to full thickness wounds • Supports autolytic debridement • Roping for tunneling • Provides odor control	• Not for dry wound bed or light exudate • Not for wounds with stable eschar • Change every 1-2 days • Requires secondary dressing • Irrigate wound between dressing changes to remove any remaining alginate
MODERATE TO HEAVY EXUDATE	**Foam:** • Non-adherent, absorptive, polyurethane • Available with silver for infection *Brands: Allevyn, Biatain, Hydrocell, PolyMem*	• Moderate to heavy exudate • Partial or full thickness wounds with moist necrosis • Good for deep/cavitating wounds • Change daily if using on infected wounds • May use around tubes	• Not for dry wound bed or light exudate • Not for wounds with stable eschar • Change every 1-4 days depending on amount of drainage • Some foam products require secondary dressing, such as gauze, to secure to fragile skin • May use as secondary dressing • Can cause maceration if not changed regularly.

Chart content adapted from:

• Burghardt JC, Robinson JM, Tscheschlog BA, Bartelmo JM. *Wound Care Made Incredibly Visual.* 2nd ed. Philadelphia:Lippincott Williams Wilkins © 2012

• Bryant RA, Nix DP, eds. *Acute & Chronic Wounds: Current Management Concepts.* 4th ed. St Louis, MO:Elsevier/Mosby. © 2012

Debridement

DEBRIDEMENT: Removal of necrotic tissue and debris from a wound. Debridement is indicated for any wound, acute or chronic, when necrotic tissue or foreign bodies are present or when the wound is infected. [1,2] While debridement is a requirement for wound healing, and therefore often regarded as an aggressive intervention, the patient's quality of life is also likely to be impacted if a wound is not debrided. The benefits of debridement for the patient at the end of life include less wound exudate and less frequent dressing changes, decreased wound odor, and reduced wound bioburden leading to lower risk of wound infection. Even if healing is not the goal of wound care, debridement allows visualization of the wound bed, and interrupts the cycle of chronic wounds to more closely resemble an acute healable wound. If necrotic tissue is present in the form of slough or eschar, the question should not be IF debridement is appropriate, but what TYPE of debridement is appropriate and in line with the patient's goals of care. Debridement is discontinued when the wound bed is clean and viable tissue is present. Arterial ulcers should not be debrided unless the blood supply is known. Also, debridement is not indicated for:

- Dry, stable (non-infected) ischemic wounds
- Wounds with dry gangrene
- Stable eschar covered heels

More Common Types of Debridement in Hospice and End of Life Care

Types of Debridement	Description
AUTOLYTIC	• Use of semi-occlusive hydrocolloid, hydrogel, or transparent dressings to keep wound bed moist, or eschar wet until it liquefies. Autolysis is a natural, painless method of debridement. Autolysis is not recommended as the sole method of debridement in infected wounds, wounds with necrotic tissue, or in the presence of significant tunneling or undermining. [1,2]
CHEMICAL	• **Enzymatic:** Uses enzymes from plants in combination with urea to digest proteins in necrotic tissue. [4] Collagenase (Santyl®) is the only enzymatic debriding agent approved in the U.S. Collagenase is derived from *Clostridium* bacteria and digests necrotic tissue by dissolving the collagen securing avascular tissue to the wound bed. Enzymes may be used to debride a wound with bacterial bioburden or infection. Silver dressings and cadexomer iodine inactivate collagenase – do not use these dressing concurrently. A secondary dressing is required over collagenase. Change dressings once or twice per day. [1] Note: Trypsin, Balsam Peru & Castor oil (Granulex®, Xenaderm®) are not effective for debriding, but may be used as a protectant on stage 1 or 2 pressure ulcers.
	• **Dakin's® solution:** (sodium hypochlorite) can be used as a chemical debriding agent as a wet-to-moist dressing. By moistening the hypochlorite soaked gauze prior to removal from the wound, viable tissue is not damaged and the process is not painful for the patient. The chemical action of the hypochlorite results in denaturing of protein to loosen slough for easier removal from the wound bed. Full strength solution (0.5%) results in partial to complete degradation of collagen. If debridement is the goal, the dressing is changed twice daily. Dilute hypochlorite solutions [half-strength (0.25%) or quarter-strength (0.125%)] can be used fewer than 10 days as an antimicrobial agent. However, once infection & odor are under control & viable tissue exposed, an alternative dressing & debridement technique should be implemented. [1]

40

Less Common Types of Debridement in Hospice and End of Life Care

Types of Debridement	Description
BIOSURGICAL	• Using therapeutic larval therapy (maggots) to remove necrotic tissue. Larvae secrete proteolytic enzymes rapidly breaking down necrotic tissue. Microorganisms are also ingested by the larvae. Some patients may not be comfortable with the sensation of crawling or movement in the wound. Nylon netting may be used to contain the larvae. Larval therapy should not be used for wounds that are poorly perfused, have exposed blood vessels, or necrotic bone. Possible treatment of choice for wet gangrene.[3]
MECHANICAL	• Non-selective, physical removal of non-viable tissue and surface debris using dressings, irrigation, or hydrotherapy. • Wet-to-dry gauze dressings & irrigation to separate necrotic tissue from the wound. Mechanical debridement is painful and may damage newly formed viable tissue. Frequent dressing changes (3 to 6 times/day) are required for several days to weeks. Not usually recommended in palliative care. Other techniques of mechanical debridement include whirlpool and pulsed lavage.
SHARP/SURGICAL	• A rapid process using sterile instruments. Conservative sharp debridement removes loosely adherent, nonviable tissue using sterile instruments (e.g. forceps, scissors, and scalpel). Surgical sharp debridement is the fastest method of removing large amounts of necrotic tissue. Surgical debridement removes necrotic tissue, eliminates bacterial bioburden, and may include techniques to reduce bleeding. The surgical process can convert a chronic wound to an acute, healable wound. Any method of sharp debridement must be done by trained and licensed health care professionals.[1] • Surgical debridement is usually avoided, but is an option if compatible with the patient's palliative goals of care.[1]

References Chapter 8

1. Ramundo J. Wound debridement. In Bryant RA, Nix DP, eds. *Acute & Chronic Wounds: Current Management Concepts.* 4th ed. St Louis, MO:Elsevier/Mosby. © 2012, p279-288

2. Lippincott, Williams and Wilkins. Wound Care Made Incredibly Visual.[2nd] Edition

3. Tippett A. How does biotherapy relate to wound care? WoundSource.com. January 2012. [Internet] Available from: http://www.woundsource.com/blog/how-does-biotherapy-relate-wound-care. Accessed 6/6/2012

4. Krasner DL, Rodeheaver GT, Sibbald RG. Interprofessional wound caring. In Krasner DL, Rodeheaver GT, Sibbald RG, eds. *Chronic Wound Care: A Clinical Sourcebook for Healthcare Professionals.* 4th ed. Malvern, PA: HMP Communications. ©2007, p.3-9

Wound Care Products

Wound Products Chart

Product & Description	Indications	Comments
Alginates: • Calcium alginate has hemostatic activity • Silver alginate has antimicrobial activity • Derived from brown seaweed • Absorbs serous fluid to form gel mass that conforms to the shape of the wound • Available in sheets or ropes; cut to the size of wound or packed into dead space • *Brands: Algisite, Aquacel, Kaltostat, Maxorb, Medihoney, Restore Calcicare, Silvercel*	Appropriate for: • moderate to heavy exudate • partial or full-thickness wound • Promotes autolytic debridement • Fibers encourage hemostasis in minimally bleeding wounds • May be layered for more absorption	• Do not use in dry wounds or wounds covered with eschar • Never use with hydrogels • Hydrofibers (Aquacel®), or fibergels, have some properties of alginates but are not hemostatic and are non-wicking; fibers provide stability for packing • Change every 1-3 days • Always requires secondary dressing
Antimicrobials: • Inhibit the growth of bacteria • Available in many forms: creams, ointments, irrigation solutions, impregnated dressings, cleansing solutions • Dressings contain silver, iodine, or polyhexanide available in various forms: transparent dressings, foams, absorptive fillers • *Dressing Brands: Acticoat, Arglaes Powder, Biatain, Maxorb Ag, Mepilex Ag, SilvaSorb, Medihoney* • *Solutions: Acetic acid, chlorhexidine, hydrogen peroxide, povidone-iodine, Dakin's solution* • *Ointment/Cream/Gels: Honey, mupirocin ointment, metronidazole: gel or crushed tablets*	• Silver based dressings inhibit bacterial growth and are effective on aerobic, anaerobic, gram-negative, gram-positive, yeast, filamentous fungi & viruses; resistance to silver is very rare • Metronidazole gel or crushed tablets can be used in combination with calcium alginate or foam dressings reducing bacterial load at the wound site and eliminating odor in 3-7 days • Honey produces hydrogen peroxide, has anti-inflammatory properties; formulated into gels or pre-impregnated pads or alginates	• Honey is contraindicated in patients with a hypersensitivity to honey. Patients with bee sting allergies are allergic to bee venom and will not be affected by the honey. Do not use in dry, necrotic wounds. (See additional information on honey, Other Therapies, page 51) • Silver-based dressings will not improve cellulitis
Collagen Products: • Collagen protein is degraded in chronic wounds; collagen dressings are derived from bovine, porcine or avian (cow, pig, or bird) sources • Informed consent or discussion of use of animal-sourced dressings. Use of some products may be refused by Muslim, Jewish, & Hindu populations[1] • May also contain silver to provide antimicrobial properties • Available as gels, alginates, sheets, or powders • *Brands: Biostep Ag Collagen Matrix, Promogran*	Appropriate for: • minimal to moderate exudate • full-thickness wounds • wounds with tunneling • chronic, granulated wounds • Wound healing stimulated by deposit of collagen fibers needed for tissue and blood vessel growth • Hemostatic properties	• Contraindicated in patients with sensitivity to collagen, bovine, porcine or avian products • Requires secondary dressing • Do not use with dry wound bed • Treat wound for infection & debride necrotic tissue before using collagen dressing • Pressure ulcer guidelines (NPUAP-EPUAP) recommend use of collagen dressings for non-healing Stage 3 & 4 pressure ulcers. • Collagen dressings are more expensive & time consuming to apply than hydrocolloid dressings

Wound Products Chart

Product & Description	Indications	Comments
Composite Dressings: • Combine physically distinct dressing components into single dressings with multiple functions • *Brands: Covrsite Plus, Stratsorb, TelfaPlus Barrier Island Dressing*	Appropriate for: • dry to heavy exudate • partial or full-thickness wound • wound with or without depth • wounds with granulation or necrotic tissue • Promotes autolytic debridement	• Functions as primary or secondary dressing • May use with topical medications: silver sulfadiazine, honey, or metronidazole
Contact Layers/Silicone Dressings: • Porous, non-adherent, silicone mesh sheets; woven or perforated for placement over the wound bed; fluid passes through for absorption into separate dressing • Contact layer stays in place during dressing changes, protecting the wound bed from trauma; easily removed – do not traumatize the wound or surrounding skin • *Brands: Mepitel Wound Contact layer, Profore Wound Contact Layer, Restore Contact Layer, Tegaderm non-adherent Contact Layer*	Appropriate for: • partial or full-thickness wounds • wound with or without depth • infected wounds; may apply topical agent over contact layer	• Not recommended for dry wounds; wounds with thick, viscous exudates; wounds with tunneling or undermining • Change weekly; not intended to be changed with each dressing change

Debridement:
• Removal of nonviable tissue from a wound
• Reduces bioburden, controls infection, facilitates visualization of the wound base
• Types of debridement: autolytic, biosurgical, chemical/enzymatic, mechanical, sharp
	Appropriate for:
	• Any wound, acute or chronic, when necrotic tissue, foreign bodies, or infection present
	• See Types of Debridement, page 40 and specific wound treatment grids for more information
		• Discontinue debridement when wound bed is clean and viable tissue is present
		• Debridement *not* indicated for:
		  • Dry, stable (non-infected) ischemic wounds
		  • Wounds with dry gangrene
		  • Stable eschar covered heels

Foam: • Absorbent, sponge-like polymer dressings; create moist wound environment, provide comfort, allow moisture to evaporate, wick drainage away from wound, allow trauma-free removal of dressing • Available with silver • *Brands: Allevyn, Biatain Foam, Mepilex, Optifoam, PolyMem, Restore Foam*	Appropriate for: • moderate to heavy exudate • partial or full thickness wounds • wounds with or without depth • venous ulcers • around drainage tubes	• Do not use on ischemic wound with dry eschar • May apply topical agent or primary dressing to wound base • Pre-shaped dressings available to fit the heel, elbow, sacrum, ear or nose • Change every 3-7 days and as needed • Available as adherent or non-adherent so may or may not require secondary dressing to secure
Gauze: • Available as woven or non-woven, cotton or synthetic, sterile or non-sterile; in many forms (pads, ribbon, strips and roll); plain or impregnated.	Appropriate for: • Securing a dressing • Gentle wound cleansing • Low cost and versatile	• Moisture evaporates quickly; drying of dressing results in painful removal and removal of healthy tissue • Frequent dressing changes required; increased patient discomfort and increased caregiver time • Associated with increased infection rates; increased costs for antimicrobials and slower healing rates

43

Wound Products Chart

Product & Description	Indications	Comments

Honey:
• Manuka (*Leptospermum*) honey is derived from the tea tree. Medical grade honey is purified for medical use with filtration & radiation
• Available as calcium alginate, hydrocolloid, paste, gel
• *Brand: MediHoney*
	Appropriate for:
	  • partial or full-thickness wounds
	  • venous, arterial & pressure ulcers
	  • wounds with tunneling or undermining
	• Reduces pain, inflammation, edema, exudate, and scarring
	• Reduces odor
	• Promotes autolytic debridement
		• Contraindicated: hypersensitivity to honey
		• Patients with bee sting allergies are allergic to bee venom and will not be affected by the honey
		• Not recommended for dry, necrotic wounds; following incision & drainage of an abscess; wounds requiring surgical debridement

Hydrocolloids:
• Occlusive & adhesive wafer dressings; react with wound exudate to form gel-like covering protecting the wound bed, maintains moist wound environment.
• Available as wafer, powder, paste
• *Brands: Duoderm, Exuderm, Replicare*
	Appropriate for:
	  • light to moderate exudates
	  • partial to full-thickness wounds
	  • superficial wounds
	• Promotes autolytic debridement
	• Can be used to frame a wound requiring frequent dressing changes; secure with tape to protect surrounding skin
		• Use on wounds with depth only as a secondary dressing
		• Impermeable to external contaminates, reducing infection risk
		• Molds to body contour
		• Contraindicated on wounds with sinus tracts, tunneling
		• Avoid use on infected wound or dry eschar
		• Use skin protectant on fragile periwound skin
		• Change every 3-5 days
		• May have odor when removed—not an indication of infection.

Hydrogel:
• Glycerin- or water-based polymers that are primarily designed to donate moisture to the wound, thus facilitating moist wound healing.
• Available as sheet, amorphous gel, or impregnated gauze
• *Brands: Skintegrity, Elasto-Gel, Vigilon*
	Appropriate for:
	  • wounds with minimal or no exudate
	  • partial or full thickness wound
	  • malignant wound
	  • wound with fungal infection & pruritus
	• Cool sheets in refrigerator to relieve pruritus
	• Promotes autolytic debridement
	• Decreases pain; cool & soothing
		• Change sterile gel dressing every 3 days
		• Change non-sterile gel dressing daily
		• Do NOT use as a wound filler
		• Requires secondary dressing
		• Softens necrotic tissue
		• Protect periwound tissue from maceration with skin sealant

Skin Barrier Film: • Liquid skin protectors protect vulnerable or fragile skin from mechanical or chemical injury, excessive moisture due to incontinence, perspiration, or wound drainage • Transparent protective coating forms on the skin • Available as foam applicator, disposable wipes, spray bottle, unit dose • *Brands: Cavilon No Sting Barrier Film, No Sting Skin Prep, Sure Prep-No Sting, Granulex, Xenaderm*	Appropriate for: • Stage I & 2 pressure ulcers • Pressure points and bony prominences • Under adhesive products to protect skin • Skin protection around stomas	• Some products contain alcohol (may cause burning sensation on open areas) • Also known as "skin sealant" • Alcohol free products: Cavilon No Sting®, No Sting Skin Prep®, Sure Prep-No Sting®

44

Wound Products Chart

Product & Description	Indications	Comments

Transparent Film:
• Semi-permeable membrane; waterproof yet permeable to water & oxygen
• No absorption capacity; impermeable to fluids & bacteria
• *Brands: Mepore, Opsite, Suresite, Tegaderm*
	Appropriate for:
	  • dry to minimal exudate
	  • partial-thickness wound
	  • eschar to promote autolytic debridement
	• Promotes autolytic debridement
	• Reduces friction
	• Use as primary or secondary dressing
		• Purulent-appearing fluid may collect under the film but is not indicative of infection.
		• Contraindicated: acutely infected wound; arterial ulcers
		• Skin sealant recommended to protect periwound tissue
		• Change dressing every 3-7 days
		• Not for wounds with depth, undermining or tunneling

Wound Cleanser: • Every open wound requires cleansing with each dressing change to physically remove surface bacteria & debris • *Brands: Allclenz, Carraklenz, Skintegrity.* Irrigate with 4-15 psi: • Spray bottle: 1.2 psi • Piston syringe: 4.2 psi • Squeeze bottle with irrigation cap: 4.5 psi • 35 mL syringe and 18 gauge needle: 8 psi • Proper sharps precautions required if using this method	**Types of Cleansers:** • **Normal Saline:** wound cleanser of choice in hospitals; does not contain preservative- use fresh solution daily to prevent bacterial contamination • **Commercially prepared cleansers:** contain surfactants which loosen and lift debris; follow product specific expiration dating **Antimicrobial Cleansers:** • Acetic Acid 0.5-5%: activity against *Pseudomonas* • Chlorhexidine: activity against Gram (+) & Gram (-) bacteria • Hydrogen Peroxide: provides mechanical debridement • Povidone-iodine: broad spectrum antimicrobial • Sodium hypochlorite (Dakin's® solution): activity against Gram (-) bacteria, MRSA	• Rinse wound bed with normal saline after cleansing with antimicrobials to minimize toxic effects **Product (Commercially Available Concentrations)** • Acetic Acid (0.5, 5%) • Chlorhexidine (4%): Must be diluted. • Hydrogen Peroxide: Often used half strength; avoid in sinus tracts due to risk of air embolism • Povidone-iodine (5, 7.5, 10, 15%): may dry and stain skin; toxic with prolonged use or over large areas; use caution in patients with burns, renal insufficiency, and thyroid disorders • Sodium hypochlorite (Dakin's® solution 0.5% full, 0.25% half, 0.125% quarter, 0.0125% Di-Dak-Sol®): Slightly dissolves necrotic tissue; If not commercially prepared, unused solution must be discarded after 24 hours

Wound Filler:
• Dressing materials placed into open wounds to eliminate dead space, absorb exudate, or maintain moisture
• Available forms:
  • hydrated (pastes, gels)
  • dry (powder, granules, beads)
  • other (ropes spiral, pillows)
• *Brands: Duoderm Hydroactive Paste, PolyMem Wic Silver Rope, FLEXIGEL Strands.*
	Appropriate for:
	  • minimal to moderate exudates
	  • full-thickness wounds with depth
	  • infected or non-infected wound
	  • wounds with dead space
		• Use appropriate secondary dressing to optimize moist wound environment.
		• Change dressing every 1-2 days
		• Contraindicated for dry wounds

Chart content adapted from:

• Burghardt JC, Robinson JM, Tscheschlog BA, Bartelmo JM. *Wound Care Made Incredibly Visual.* 2nd ed. Philadelphia:Lippincott Williams Wilkins © 2012
• Bryant RA, Nix DP, eds. *Acute & Chronic Wounds: Current Management Concepts.* 4th ed. St Louis, MO:Elsevier/Mosby. © 2012
• Wounds 360. Ostomy Wound Management (OWM) Online Buyers Guide. [Internet] Available from: http://www.wounds360bg.com/ Accessed 6/6/2012

Topical Medicated Agents for Skin & Wound Care[2]

Medication	Brand Examples	Dosage Forms	Cost (Amt)*	Comments
Anesthetics				
Lidocaine	Xylocaine®	Cream, ointment, Gel, Solution	$ (100mL)	Viscous lidocaine 2% is recommended
Lidocaine 2.5% -Prilocaine 2.5%	EMLA®	Cream	$$ (30g)	Avoid application to open wounds
Antimicrobials				
Bacitracin	Baciguent®	Ointment	$ (15g)	Active against Gram+ bacilli.
Bacitracin & Polymyxin B	Polysporin®	Ointment, powder	$ (15g)	Risk of contact dermatitis with use developing over several days; anaphylaxis is rare but occurs rapidly after exposure
Bacitracin, Polymyxin B, Neomycin	Neosporin®	Ointment	$ (15g)	
Cadexomer iodine	Iodosorb®	Gel, ointment, tincture	$$$ (40g)	Broad spectrum germicidal against virus, bacteria, spores, fungi, protozoa
Gentian violet	n/a	Solution	$ (100mL)	Has antifungal and antimicrobial properties
Honey (*Leptospermum*)	Medihoney®	Gel, paste	$$ (44g)	Broad spectrum antibacterial activity. Contraindicated if hypersensitivity to honey.
Metronidazole 1% or 0.75% (*Metronidazole 1% is brand only*)	Metrogel 1%®	Gel	$$$ (0.75%) $$$$ (1%)	Crushing oral tablets and applying to wounds for odor control is more cost effective than commercial metronidazole gels.
Mupirocin	Bactroban® , Centany®	Cream, ointment	$$ (22g)	Active against MRSA, MSSA, *S. pyogenes*
Silver sulfadiazine	Silvadene®	Ointment	$ (25g)	Avoid use if sulfonamide allergy. Broad spectrum bactericidal activity.
Antifungals				
Clotrimazole	Lotrimin®	Cream, solution	$$ (30g)	Available with betamethasone as Lotrisone
Ketoconazole	Extina 2%®, Xolegel 2%®	Cream, foam, gel	$$ (30g)	Prescription gel & foam: $$$$
Miconazole	Micatin®, Monostat®	Cream, ointment, powder, spray	$$ (45g)	Available with zinc oxide as Baza AF
Nystatin	Nystop®, Pedi-dri®	Cream, ointment, powder	$$ (15g)	Available with triamcinolone as Mycolog-II: $$$$
Barriers				
Trypsin, Balsam Peru, Castor oil	Xenaderm®, Granulex®	Ointment, spray	$$ (56.7g)	Not effective for debridement, mild antibacterial
Vitamin A+D	Sween®, A+D®, Baza clear®	Cream, ointment	$ (113g)	Do not use on severe burns or deep wounds
Zinc oxide	Desitin®, Balmex®	Cream, ointment, paste, powder	$ (113g)	Available with miconazole as Baza AF
Corticosteroids				
Betamethasone	Celestone®, Diprolene®	Cream, gel, lotion, ointment	$$$$ (50g)	For all topical corticosteroids: reassess use if no improvement within 14 days
Clobetasol	Clobex®, Temovate®	Cream, foam, gel, lotion, ointment	$$$ (30g)	Betamethasone+clotrimazole as Lotrisone: $$$
Fluocinonide	Lidex®, Vanos®	Cream, gel, ointment	$$ (30g)	Triamcinolone+nystatin as Mycolog-II: $$$$
Fluocinolone	Derma-smoothe®	Cream, oil, ointment	$$ (15g)	
Hydrocortisone	Cortizone®, Cortaid®	Cream, foam, gel, ointment	$ (15g)	
Triamcinolone	Kenalog®, Triderm®	Cream, lotion, ointment, spray	$$ (15g)	
Debriders				
Collagenase	Santyl®	Ointment	$$$ (30g)	Will not affect healthy tissue, fat, fibrin, keratin, or muscle

- Average Cost per Package as of January 2013: $ = <$10, $$ = $11-50, $$$ = $51-100, $$$$ = >$100

Recipes for Wound Care Preparations

Wound Prep	Components*	Comments
Diluted hypochlorite solution (Dakin's®)[3] ¼ strength (0.125%) ½ strength (0.25%)	Household bleach (sodium hypochlorite 5.25%) <ul><li>½ strength: 25mL (1T+2 tsp)</li><li>¼ strength: 12.5mL (2 ½ tsp)</li></ul> Baking soda: ½ tsp 32 oz boiled tap water, cooled 32 oz container, sterile *Directions:* Boil tap water, cool. Add ½ tsp baking soda (buffering agent) and amount of bleach for desired strength solution. Stir to dissolve and transfer to sterile container.	<ul><li>Dispose of any unused solution within 24 hours</li><li>Use only unscented, regular strength bleach (Clorox®)</li><li>Dakin's solution is a commercially available wound cleansing product with published stability information; however, the stability and sterility of compounded hypochlorite solution cannot be guaranteed.</li><li>Short term use only (less than 14 days).</li></ul>
Acetic acid irrigation solution[3,4] 0.25%	Distilled white vinegar <ul><li>0.25%: 50mL (3T + 1 tsp)</li></ul> 32 oz boiled tap water, cooled 32 oz container, sterile *Directions:* Boil tap water, cool. Add 50mL vinegar. Stir solution well and transfer to sterile container.	<ul><li>Dispose of any unused solution within 24 hours</li><li>Acetic acid irrigation solution is a commercially available cleansing product with published stability information; however, the stability and sterility of compounded acetic acid solution cannot be guaranteed.</li><li>May have anti-*Pseudomonas* activity</li><li>Short term use only (less than 14 days).</li></ul>
Morphine in hydrogel[5]	Morphine for injection (10mg/mL): 10mg (1mL) Hydrogel (Intrasite): 8g Apply 5-10mL to wound and cover with dressing May be applied 1 to 3 times per day	<ul><li>Painful open wounds</li><li>No benefit if skin is intact (stage 1 pressure ulcer)</li><li>No systemic analgesic effect from topical application</li><li>Pharmacist-prepared compounded product is stable under controlled room temperature for 28 days.[6]</li></ul>
Morphine topical solution[7]	Morphine for injection (10mg/mL): 20mg (2mL) Normal saline: 8mL Creates 0.2% morphine solution to be used as a topical spray for painful open wounds. *Alternate formulation:* Morphine 4%+Lidocaine 4% topical spray with each dressing change	<ul><li>Painful open wounds</li><li>No benefit if skin is intact (stage 1 pressure ulcer)</li><li>No systemic analgesic effect</li><li>Pharmacist-prepared compounded product is stable under controlled room temperature for 14 days.</li><li>Larger volumes may also be compounded</li></ul>
Metronidazole topical solution[8]	Metronidazole (Flagyl®) tablet (500mg): 1000mg Normal saline: 100mL Crush tablets and dissolve in 100mL of normal saline to create 1% solution. Use as irrigation solution with dressing changes.	<ul><li>To reduce odor only; will not treat wound infection</li><li>Metronidazole topical solution may be prepared at bedside; discard any unused solution after each treatment</li><li>Metronidazole topical solution may be more effective to use for wounds with tunneling where powder from crushed tablets will not sufficiently reach</li></ul>

*Boil tap water 20 minutes and cool to room temperature. Prepare clean containers by boiling or sanitizing in dishwasher. Follow your organizations' policy for clean vs sterile preparation.[3]

References Chapter 9

1. Enoch S, Shaaban H, Dunn KW. Informed consent should be obtained from patients to use products (skin substitutes) and dressings containing biological material. *J Med Ethics* 2005;31:2-6

2. Lexi-Comp Online, Lexi-Drugs Online, Hudson, Ohio: Lexi-Comp, Inc.; June 6, 2013

3. Brown P. Quick reference to wound care. 4th ed. Burlington, MA: Jones & Bartlett Learning; c2012. Chapter 4 Basics of wound management; p. 25-40

4. Drosou A, Falabella A, Kirsner RS. Antiseptics on wounds: an area of controversy. Wounds 2008. [Internet] Available from: http://www.woundsresearch.com/article/1586

5. Tran QNH, Fancher T. Achieving analgesia for painful ulcers using topically applied morphine gel. *J Support Oncol* 2007;5(6):289-293

6. Zeppetella G, Joel SP, Ribeiro MDC. Stability of morphine sulphate and diamorphine hydrochloride in Intrasite gel. *Palliat Med* 2005;19:131-136

7. Jacobson J. Topical opioids for pain. *Fast Facts and Concepts* 2007; 184. [Internet] Available from: http://www.eperc.mcw.edu/fastfact/ff_184.htm

8. Zip CM. Innovative use of topical metronidazole. *Dermatol Clin* 2010;28(3):525-534

9. Burghardt JC, Robinson JM, Tscheschlog BA, Bartelmo JM. *Wound Care Made Incredibly Visual.* 2nd ed. Philadelphia:Lippincott Williams Wilkins © 2012

10. Bryant RA, Nix DP, eds. *Acute & Chronic Wounds: Current Management Concepts.* 4th ed. St Louis, MO:Elsevier/Mosby. © 2012

11. Wounds 360. Ostomy Wound Management (OWM) Online Buyers Guide. [Internet] Available from: http://www.wounds360bg.com/ Accessed 6/6/2012

48

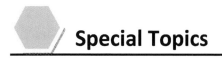

Skin Tears[1,2]

Skin tears are traumatic injuries to the skin of older adults, primarily on the extremities. Shearing and friction forces cause the separation of skin layers (epidermis from dermis). Skin tears may be partial or full thickness depending on the degree of damage to skin tissue. Skin tears are associated with many risk factors, including age >75 years, immobility, long-term corticosteroid use, inadequate nutrition, impaired cognitive status, neuropathy, dependence on activities of daily living, etc. A 2011 survey found the top causes of skin tears: blunt trauma, falls, performing activities of daily living (ADLs), dressing/treatment related, patient transfer (friction and shear), and equipment injury. Skin tears should be assessed and documented routinely and a skin tear may be reclassified as a pressure ulcer if pressure, shear and friction are the underlying cause. Treatment is aimed at preserving the remaining skin flap, protecting the surrounding tissue, and closing the edges of the wound, thereby reducing the risk of infection and further injury. Cleanse the wound with warm saline or water. Select an appropriate dressing; a moist wound environment tends to enhance and accelerate wound healing. Steri-strips may be appropriate with careful use to avoid further damage. Dressings should be secured using a non-adhesive product: stockinet sleeves, gauze, or self-adhering tape (Coban®).

Deep Tissue Injury[3]

Deep tissue injury (DTI) is a form of pressure ulcer defined by the NPUAP as a "pressure-related injury to subcutaneous tissues under intact skin." Because the extent of injury is not known, DTI may be considered unstageable. DTI appear initially as a deep bruise but may rapidly deteriorate into stage 3 or 4 pressure ulcers despite optimal care. Although pressure offloading and symptomatic treatment should be attempted, treatments may not prevent further deterioration. Consider the differential diagnoses of regular healable bruises, calciphylaxis, hematoma, gangrene, and abscess. The NPUAP recommends developing nomenclature and staging systems to specifically address DTI, separate from the pressure ulcer staging system.

Calciphylaxis[3,4]

Calciphylaxis is vascular calcification and skin necrosis most common in patients with a long-standing history of chronic renal failure and dialysis. The only recognized non-uremic cause of calciphylaxis is primary hyperparathyroidism. Lesions may be bluish-purple, tender, and extremely firm. Lesions are commonly seen on the lower extremities, not bony prominences. The incidence of these lesions is very low in general (non-ESRD) patient populations. Calciphylaxis should be suspected in patients with painful, non-ulcerated subcutaneous nodules, non-healing ulcers, or necrosis. These should not be debrided. Warfarin, corticosteroids, calcium-based binders, and vitamin D analogs may increase the risk of calciphylaxis. For patients on warfarin therapy, risks and benefits should be considered as warfarin may increase the risk of progression of non-healing necrotic ulcers. Calciphylaxis signals a poor prognosis for patients with ESRD.

Kennedy Terminal Ulcers[5]

Kennedy Terminal Ulcers (KTU) are a subgroup of pressure ulcers that develop rapidly in patients who are close to death. Initial appearance may resemble an abrasion, blister, or darkened area, but the wound will rapidly progress to a stage 2, 3, or 4 pressure ulcer. KTUs are typically in the shape of a pear, butterfly or horseshoe with irregular edges. Color quickly changes from red to yellow to black. KTUs are most often seen on the sacrum or coccyx but can be found over any bony prominence. Skin is the largest organ of the body and is subject to the effects of the dying process. KTUs may be a result of decreased tissue perfusion, in addition to decreased tolerance of pressure and incontinence. Compromised immune response due to the administration of corticosteroids or immunosuppressants may also increase risk. Treatment of a Kennedy Terminal Ulcer is determined by the stage of the ulcer. All areas of treatment need to be addressed and treated accordingly: cleansing, dressing, infection, pain, and support surface. Despite appropriate interventions, these ulcers cannot heal.

References Chapter 10

1. Bryant RA. Types of skin damage and differential diagnosis. In Bryant RA, Nix DP, eds. *Acute & Chronic Wounds: Current Management Concepts.* 4th ed. St Louis, MO:Elsevier/Mosby. © 2012, p83-107

2. LeBlanc K, Baranoski S, Skin Tear Consensus Panel Members. Skin tears: state of the science: consensus statements for the prevention, prediction, assessment, and treatment of skin tears. *Adv Skin Wound Care* 2012;24(9suppl):2-15

3. National Pressure Ulcer Advisory Panel. NPUAP White Paper [Internet]. Deep tissue injury. 2012. [Internet] Available from: http://www.npuap.org/wp-content/uploads/2012/01/DTI-White-Paper.pdf

4. Santos PW, Hartle JE, Quarles LD. Calciphylaxis. In UpToDate, Goldfarb S. (Ed) UpToDate, Waltham, MA, 2012

5. Kennedy-Evans K. Understanding the Kennedy terminal ulcer. *Ostomy Wound Manage* 2009;55(9):6

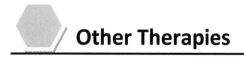

Other Therapies

Evidence-based information is the foundation of choosing any treatment, including an evaluation of treatment efficacy and safety. The clinician must be aware of less traditional interventions, including cultural preferences that may contribute to patient comfort and quality of life. However, the same critical thinking and evidence-based practice that proves successful in other areas of patient care must also be utilized when considering non-conventional treatments.

BIOTHERAPY:

Biotherapy uses living creatures for diagnosis or treatment of human disease. Common modalities include larvae (maggots), leeches, honey bees, and viruses. Honey and larval therapy are increasingly recognized as useful treatments in wound care.[1]

Honey:

Honey has been used for wound treatment dating back to ancient Egyptians and Greeks.[2] Recent studies have found that honey has an inhibitory effect on up to 60 species of bacteria, aerobic and anaerobic, Gram-positive and Gram-negative. Antifungal action has also been observed for some yeast and species of *Aspergillus* and *Penicillium*.[3] *Leptospermum* (Manuka or tea tree) honey, has an inhibitory effect on *Pseudomonas aeruginosa*, methicillin-resistant *S. aureus* (MRSA), and vancomycin-resistant enterococcus (VRE).[2]

Honey's ability to aid in wound healing and treat infections can be linked to various mechanisms of action. Honey contains glucose oxidase, an enzyme that converts glucose to hydrogen peroxide, an anti-microbial agent.[2] However, hydrogen peroxide concentration in honey is approximately 1000 times less than that found in the 3% hydrogen peroxide solutions commonly used as an antiseptic, thus avoiding tissue damage.[3] Medical grade honey is filtered, gamma-irradiated, and produced under carefully controlled standards, but is more expensive. Raw or unpasteurized honey as an alternative to medical grade honey has been studied and used in various types of wounds. Honey's therapeutic value can vary and is influenced by the flower source, weather, and climatic conditions.[4] Adverse reactions to honey are rare but may be caused by residual pollen. Medical grade honey used in wound care has most of the pollen removed via filtration. Some patients may report a mild stinging sensation during initial application, but not severe enough to stop treatment.[3]

Therapeutic benefits of honey:[4]
- Wound bed preparation
- Reduction of exudates due to its anti-inflammatory properties
- Facilitates autolytic debridement and consequently treatment of odor
- Reduces risk of maceration
- Management of antibiotic-resistant bacteria
- Prevention of biofilm production
- Prevention of cross-contamination

Larvae Therapy: [1,5,6]

In some countries, larval therapy with maggots is the standard of care for non-healing wounds. Use of larval therapy with medical maggots for wounds is uncommon in the U.S. However, maggots are highly effective for debridement and can eliminate infected and necrotic tissue without harming healthy tissue. Growth factors and enzymes secreted by the maggots also seem to assist in wound healing.[1] Not all fly maggots can be used for larval therapy. Medical maggots are an FDA-approved medical device for wound debridement. Medical maggots will only feed on necrotic tissue. Sterile medical maggots can be purchased from Monarch Labs. Additional information is Available from: http://www.monarchlabs.com.

Larval therapy wound care may be considered: [1,5,6]

- When sharp debridement is difficult due to exposed bone, joint, or tendon
- When autolytic debridement attempts have failed
- As a follow-up method of debridement after sharp debridement
- For necrotic or gangrenous wounds
- For debilitated patients who cannot tolerate antibiotics

Maggots can debride an open, necrotic wound, removing bacteria in 24-72 hours. An average larval therapy application consumes 10 to 15 grams of necrotic tissue each day. Treatment consists of a base dressing (nylon netting placed over the larvae and wound) and a pad placed on top of the netting to absorb exudates and liquefied tissue. Remove larvae from the wound after 3 days with a warm saline rinse. Larvae can be used in conjunction with conventional systemic antibiotic treatment.

COMPRESSION THERAPY:[7-9]
The majority of leg ulcers are due to venous insufficiency, resulting in an accumulation of blood in the legs. The main treatment has been a firm compression garment (bandage or stocking) to provide support and to aid venous return. Compression increases ulcer healing rates compared with no compression. Multi-component systems are more effective than single-component systems. Multi-component systems containing an elastic bandage appear more effective than those composed mainly of inelastic constituents.[8]

Select compression methods based on careful assessment of the patient:[9]

- Elastic component added to two and three component systems might be beneficial.
- Anti-embolism stockings or hose (15-17 mmHg) are *not* designed for therapeutic compression.
- Consider using a multi-layer system that contains an elastic layer.
- Modified, reduced compression bandaging (23-30 mmHg at the ankle) for mixed arterial/venous disease and moderate arterial insufficiency (ABI: 0.5-0.8 mmHg) for patients with ulcers and edema.
- Consider using intermittent pneumatic compression (IPC) for patients who are immobile or who need higher levels of compression than that which can be provided with stockings or wraps (i.e., those with extremely large legs or who are intolerant of stockings or wraps) or who have not responded to stockings/wrap.

NEGATIVE PRESSURE WOUND THERAPY:[10,11]
Negative pressure wound therapy (NPWT), a common brand is wound VAC™, is a controlled application of negative pressure to accelerate debridement and promote healing in wounds. Negative pressure assists with removal of interstitial fluid, decreasing localized edema, and increasing blood flow. These processes may also decrease bacterial level in tissue. Negative pressure can be delivered intermittently or continuously with optimum suction being 125 mmHg. However, the benefits of intermittent therapy may be outweighed by the potential loss of seal and subsequent backflow of wound fluid, as well as the increased caregiver supervision required to monitor intermittent therapy. Consequently, continuous therapy delivered at 125 mmHg is most routinely used.

The Agency for Healthcare Research & Quality (AHRQ) recommends NPWT as an adjuvant treatment option for stage 3 and 4 pressure ulcers. NPWT is approved for use with many wound types: chronic, acute, traumatic, sub-acute and dehisced wounds, partial-thickness burns, pressure ulcers, and diabetic ulcers. NPWT can be used for wounds with tunneling, undermining, or sinus tracts. NPWT includes a wound filler dressing, suction catheter, transparent cover dressing, suction source (i.e. pump), and collection container. Topical products (silver products, debriding agents, collagen wound dressings) may be used in conjunction with NPWT. Antimicrobial products used with NPWT may reduce the bioburden of the wound.[10,11]

Contraindications to NPWT: [10,11]
- fistulas to organs or body cavities
- necrotic tissue
- untreated osteomyelitis
- malignancy in the wound
- exposed blood vessels or organs

If the potential for hemorrhage exists NPWT can be used but with caution

The cost of NPWT is significant; in addition to the machine (pump) itself, it is necessary to purchase disposable foam dressings, drainage tubes, canisters, and adhesives drapes. This cost may cause some clinicians to be reluctant to use it. [10,11]

KETAMINE TOPICAL GELS & SOLUTIONS

Ketamine is an NMDA antagonist used as a surgical general anesthetic and as adjuvant therapy with opioids for refractory pain syndromes.[12] Topical ketamine preparations for management of neuropathic pain have limited evidence to support their use. Topical ketamine cream was not more effective than placebo in a study of use for diabetic peripheral neuropathy.[13] Frequently, topical ketamine preparations include other ingredients to boost effectiveness including amitriptyline and lidocaine.[14] Ketamine, compounded as a 5-10 mg/ml gel, may relieve pain related to postherpetic neuralgias and Reflex Sympathetic Dystrophy (RSD), as well as other neuropathic types of pain.[15,16] Ketamine mouthwash has also been used for oral mucositis pain refractory to usual "magic mouthwash" solutions (e.g., diphenhydramine, lidocaine, magnesium/aluminum hydroxide).[17,18]

LIDOCAINE TOPICAL GELS & SOLUTIONS

Lidocaine is a local anesthetic available in both injectable and topical dosage forms. Injectable lidocaine is also used as an anti-arrhythmic agent. Lidocaine reduces peripheral nociceptor sensitization by blocking sodium ion channels to prevent initiation and conduction of nerve impulses producing anesthesia.[19,20] Topical lidocaine formulations may be used to manage wound pain associated with dressing changes, debridement, or other wound care procedures.[19-23] While the risk is low, even when applied to open wounds, there is some potential for systemic absorption of lidocaine from topical application.[20-22] Larger wounds, relative to the body size of the patient, may increase the risk of systemic absorption. Due to smaller body size, increased skin permeability, and changes in fat-water distribution of subcutaneous tissue, infants and small children also have an increased risk. Some topical lidocaine products have excipients that may cause burning or irritation (e.g., ethanol, benzyl alcohol, menthol, etc). Oral topical lidocaine 2% solution, also known as viscous lidocaine, is designed specifically for mucous membrane use, lessening the risk of systemic absorption. Although clinical literature is limited on the use of viscous lidocaine 2% for use in wound care, widespread availability, ease of use, clinical experience, and anecdotal evidence indicates it is the formulation of choice. Topical EMLA® (lidocaine-prilocaine) cream has also been studied for painful wounds. EMLA® doses may range from 3g – 150g per application and is left in place for up to 60 minutes. Some patients report an uncomfortable burning sensation for several minutes after application.[23]

PHENYTOIN TOPICAL GELS & SOLUTIONS

Topical phenytoin (Dilantin®) use for acceleration of wound healing is based in the medication's ability to cause hyperplasia of gingival tissue. Phenytoin seems to stimulate collagen production and deposition in the wound and may decrease edema and bacterial load.[24] A small pilot study for treatment of chemotherapy-induced oral mucositis, results showed some improvement in pain and healing with use of topical phenytoin 0.5% oral rinse solution four times daily.[25] However, topical dressing of phenytoin in hydrogel demonstrated no benefit for diabetic foot ulcers in a randomized controlled trial.[26] Systematic review of the available literature seems to show a trend towards beneficial wound healing effects with the use of topical phenytoin. However, more data is needed before this treatment can be recommended.

References Chapter 11

1. Tippett A. How does biotherapy relate to wound care? WoundSource.com. January 2012. [Internet] Available from: http://www.woundsource.com/blog/how-does-biotherapy-relate-wound-care. Accessed 6/6/2012

2. Song JJ, Salcido R. Use of honey in wound care: an update. *Adv Skin Wound Care* 2011;24(1):40-44

3. Molan PC. Honey as topical antibacterial agent for treatment of infected wounds. December 2001. Available at http://www.worldwidewounds.com/2001/november/Molan/honey-as-topical-agent.html. Accessed 6/6/2012

4. Cutting KF. Honey and contemporary wound care: an overview. *OWM* 2007;53(11):49-54

5. Hinshaw J. Larval therapy: a review of clinical human and veterinary studies. October 2000. [Internet] Available from: http://www.worldwidewounds.com/2000/oct/Janet-Hinshaw/Larval-Therapy-Human-and-Veterinary.html. Accessed 6/6/2012

6. Sherman RA, Pechter EA. Maggot therapy: a review of the therapeutic applications of fly larvae in human medicine, especially for treating osteomylitis. *Med Vet Entomology* 1988;2(3):225-230

7. O'Meara S, Cullum NA, Nelson EA. Compression for venous leg ulcers. *Cochrane Database Syst Rev* 2009; 29(1):CD000265

8. Moffat S. Understanding compression therapy. 2003; Medical Education Partnership LTD, 2003; European Wound Management Association (EWMA). [Internet] Available from: http://www.woundsinternational.com/pdf/content_51.pdf

9. Kelechi TJ, Johnson JJ. Guideline for the management of wounds in patients with lower-extremity venous disease: an executive summary. *J Wound Ostomy Continence Nurs* 2012;39(6):598-606

10. Netsch DS. Negative pressure wound therapy. In Bryant RA, Nix DP, eds. *Acute & Chronic Wounds: Current Management Concepts.* 4th ed. St Louis, MO:Elsevier/Mosby. © 2012, p337-344

11. Gestring M, Sanfey H, Collins KA. Negative pressure wound therapy. In UpToDate, Basow DS ed. Waltham, MA. 2012.

12. Quibell R, Prommer E, Mihalyo M, Twycross R, Wilcock A. Ketamine: therapeutic review. *J Pain Symptom Manage* 2011;41(3):640-649

13. Mahoney J, Vardaxis V, Moore J, Hall A, Haffner K, Peterson M. Topical ketamine cream in the treatment of diabetic peripheral neuropathy. *J Am Podiatr Med Assoc* 2012;102(3):178-183

14. Lynch M, Clark A, Sawynok J, Sullivan M. Topical 2% amitriptyline and 1% ketamine in neuropathic pain syndromes. *Anesthesiology* 2005;103:140-6

15. Gammaitoni A, Gallagher R, Welz-Bozna M. Topical ketamine gel:possible role in treating neuropathic pain. *Pain Med* 2000;1(1):97-100

16. Quan D, Wellish M, Gilden D. Topical ketamine treatment of postherpetic neuralgia. *Neurology* 2003;60(8):1391-2

17. Slatkin N, Rhiner M. Topical ketamine in the treatment of mucositis pain. *Pain Med* 2004;4(3):298-303

18. Ryan A, Lin F, Atayee R. Ketamine mouthwash for mucositis pain. *J Palliat Med* 2009;12(11);989-91

19. Lexi-Comp Online, Lexi-Drugs Online, Hudson, Ohio: Lexi-Comp, Inc.; June 11, 2013

20. Popescu A, Salcido R. Wound pain: a challenge for the patient and the wound care specialist. *Adv Skin Wound Care* 2004;17:14-22

21. Pontani B, Feste M, Adams C, et al. Cross over clinical study of 47 patients with painful deep wounds showed use of a hydrogel containing 2% lidocaine HCl and collagen as contact layer was significant in alleviating dressing related pain. 23rd Clinical Symposium on Advances in Skin & Wound Care Oct 2008, no.30.

22. Evans E, Gray M. Do topical analgesics reduce pain associated with wound dressing changes or debridement of chronic wounds? *J Wound Ostomy Continence Nurs* 2005;32(5):287-290

23. McDonald A, Lesage P. Palliative management of pressure ulcers and malignant wounds in patients with advanced illness. *J Palliat Med* 2005;9(2):285-295

24. Shaw J, Hughes CM, Lagan KM, Bell PM. The clinical effect of topical phenytoin on wound healing: a systematic review. *Brit J Dermatol* 2007;157:997-1004

25. Baharvand M, Sarrafi M, Alavi K, Jalali ME. Efficacy of topical phenytoin on chemotherapy-induced oral mucositis: a pilot study. *DARU* 2010;18(1):46-50

26. Shaw J, Hughes CM, Lagan KM, Stevenson MR, Irwin CR, Bell PM. The effect of topical phenytoin on healing diabetic foot ulcers: a randomized controlled trial. *Diabet Med* 2011;28:1154-1157

54

Documentation

Chart documentation represents the care provided by the entire hospice clinical team. Skin assessment should be conducted and documented regularly in accordance with the policies of your organization. In the extended care setting, these assessments may be daily; while in homecare, skin assessment usually occurs with each nursing visit. Elements of wound documentation include skin assessments, wound measurements, patient repositioning schedules, utilization of support surfaces, and record of discussion with patient and caregivers about the wound care plan. When a pressure ulcer is present, charting must be thorough. Useful content includes: [1-3]

1. Dressing status: note if dressing was changed or not and its condition (e.g., intact, leakage)
2. Description of peri-ulcer area
3. Presence of possible complications: including induration, infection, or increasing ulceration
4. Pain and patient's response to analgesia
5. Description of wound appearance; specific, but do not diagnose unless you are a wound or skin specialist or physician
6. Record wound dimensions
7. Record communication with other team members and family (date, time, content of communication)
8. Document rationale for changes to the care plan; obtain orders as needed
9. Document chosen support surface

Accurate wound measurements provide support to the appropriateness of continuing a current plan of care or the need to change the plan of care. Size is determined by measuring length, width, and depth; usually in centimeters. Length and width are measured from wound edge to wound edge. Depth is measured from the visible surface to the deepest point in the wound base. Measure wounds with variable depth at different points to confirm the deepest site. Help visualize location of undermining and tunneling by using clock hour hands to symbolize position. [2] Consistently document factors contributing to impaired healing, such as disease progression, poor nutritional intake, or patient choices that interfere with healing (e.g., smoking, choosing not to turn).

In some cases wound photography may be useful. It may be used for wound assessment and diagnosis or as a method to minimize legal liability. [3] However, wound imaging does not replace the need for accurate written documentation. The Wound, Ostomy and Continence Nurses Society has developed a *Photography in Wound Documentation: Fact Sheet* which addresses issues, such as informed consent, guidelines for use of cell phones as an imaging device, and confidentiality. Information for locating this fact sheet is found in the Resource List on page 60.

Healthcare facility policies and procedures are guidelines, not rules or regulations. Problems arise when "policy" is used interchangeably with "rules" or "regulations". Avoid documentation with words such as "never,", "must," and "immediately." For example, if there is a policy that patients with a pressure ulcer "must" be turned every 2 hours, failure to do so even one time has the potential to represent a breach of the standard of care. In the event of litigation, the chart will be compared to the healthcare agency's written regulations, policies, procedures, and guidelines of the institution.

References Chapter 12

1. Ayello EA, Capitulo KL, Fowler E, Krasner DL, Mulder G, Sibbald RG, Yankowsky KW. Legal issues in the care of pressure ulcer patients: key concepts for health care providers: a consensus paper from the International Expert Wound Care Advisory Panel. *J Palliat Med* 2009;12(11):995-1008
2. Hess CT. The art of skin and wound care. *Home Healthcare Nurse* 2005;23(8):502-513
3. Brown G. Wound documentation: managing risk. *Adv Skin Wound Care* 2006;19(3):155-165

Pressure Ulcer Staging

Term	Description
Suspected deep tissue injury (depth unknown)	Purple or maroon localized area of discolored intact skin or blood-filled blister due to damage of underlying soft tissue from pressure and/or **shear.** The area may be preceded by tissue that is painful, firm, mushy, boggy, warmer or cooler as compared to adjacent tissue. Deep tissue injury may be difficult to detect in individuals with dark skin tones. Evolution may include a thin blister over a dark wound bed. The wound may further evolve and become covered by thin eschar. Evolution may be rapid, exposing additional layers of tissue even with optimal treatment.
Stage 1 Non-blanchable erythema	Intact skin with non-blanchable redness of a localized area, usually over a bony prominence. Darkly pigmented skin may not have visible blanching; its color may differ from the surrounding area. The area may be painful, firm, soft, warmer, or cooler as compared to adjacent tissue. Category I may be difficult to detect in individuals with dark skin tones. May indicate "at risk" persons.
Stage 2 Partial thickness	Partial thickness loss of dermis presenting as a shallow open ulcer with a red pink wound bed, without slough. May also present as an intact or open/ruptured serum-filled or sero-sanginous filled blister. Presents as a shiny or dry shallow ulcer without slough or bruising*. This category should not be used to describe skin tears, tape burns, incontinence associated dermatitis, maceration, or excoriation. *Bruising indicates deep tissue injury.
Stage 3 Full thickness skin loss	Full thickness tissue loss. Subcutaneous fat may be visible but bone, tendon, or muscle are *not* exposed. Slough may be present but does not obscure the depth of tissue loss. *May* include undermining and tunneling. The depth of a Category/Stage III pressure ulcer varies by anatomical location. The bridge of the nose, ear, occiput and malleolus do not have (adipose) subcutaneous tissue and Category/Stage III ulcers can be shallow. In contrast, areas of significant adiposity can develop extremely deep Category/Stage III pressure ulcers. Bone/tendon is not visible or directly palpable.
Stage 4 Full thickness tissue loss	Full thickness tissue loss with exposed bone, tendon or muscle. Slough or eschar may be present. Often includes undermining and tunneling. The depth of a Category/Stage IV pressure ulcer varies by anatomical location. The bridge of the nose, ear, occiput and malleolus do not have (adipose) subcutaneous tissue and these ulcers can be shallow. Category/Stage IV ulcers can extend into muscle and/or supporting structures (e.g., fascia, tendon or joint capsule), making osteomyelitis or osteitis likely to occur. Exposed bone/muscle is visible or directly palpable.
Unstageable Full thickness skin or tissue loss (depth unknown)	Full thickness tissue loss in which actual depth of the ulcer is completely obscured by slough (yellow, tan, gray, green or brown) and/or eschar (tan, brown or black) in the wound bed. Until enough slough and/or eschar are removed to expose the base of the wound, the true depth cannot be determined; but it will be either a Category/Stage III or IV. Stable (dry, adherent, intact without erythema or fluctuance) eschar on the heels serves as "the body's natural (biological) cover" and should not be removed.
Reverse Staging	Once layers of tissue and supporting structures are gone, such as with full-thickness wounds, they are not replaced. Instead, the wound is filled with granulation tissue. Consequently, a Stage 3 wound cannot progress to a Stage 1 or 2. A Stage 3 pressure ulcer that appears to be granulating and resurfacing is described as a healing Stage 3 pressure ulcer.

©NPUAP-EPUAP, used with permission

- National Pressure Ulcer Advisory Panel and European Pressure Ulcer Advisory Panel (NPUAP-EPUAP). NPUAP Pressure Ulcer Stages/Categories. Washington, DC: National Pressure Ulcer Advisory Panel, 2007.

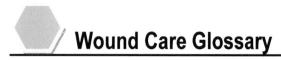

Wound Care Glossary

Term	Description
Abrasion	Wearing away of the skin through some mechanical process (friction or trauma).
Abscess	Accumulation of pus enclosed anywhere in the body.
Antibiotic	*Pharmacologic agents* that destroy or inhibit bacteria. May be broad or narrow in spectrum of activity. May be used systemically and topically.
Antifungal	*Pharmacologic agents* that inhibit the growth of fungal infections. May be broad or narrow in spectrum of activity. May be used systemically and topically.
Antimicrobial	Any agent that destroys or inhibits the growth of microbes including bacteria, fungi, viruses, or protozoa
Antiseptic	*Chemical agents* that prevent, inhibit, or destroy microorganisms including bacteria, viruses, fungi, and protozoa. Topical use only.
Autolysis	Disintegration or liquefaction of tissue or cells by the body's own mechanisms, such as leukocytes and enzymes.
Bacterial load	Total number of bacteria in a wound; may or may not cause a host response.
Bacteriostatic	Agent capable of inhibiting the growth of bacteria.
Biofilm	Polysaccharide matrix that microorganisms produce; highly resistant to antimicrobials. Must be removed by debridement.
Bioburden	Presence of microorganism on or in a wound. Continuum of bioburden ranges from contamination, colonization, critical colonization, biofilm and infection. Bioburden includes quantity of microorganism present, as well as their diversity, virulence, and interaction of the organism with each other and the body.
Blanching	Becoming white; maximum pallor
Cellulitis	Inflammation of the tissues indicating a local infection; characterized by redness, edema, and tenderness
Collagen	Main supportive protein of the skin.
Colonization	Presence of replicating bacteria that adhere to the wound bed but do not cause cellular damage to the host.
Contamination	Non-replicating microorganisms on the wound surface without a host reaction. All open wounds are contaminated by normal skin flora.
Critical colonization/Local infection	Increasing bacterial load on a wound that is between the category of colonization and infection. Wound does not heal but may not display classic signs of infection.
Dead space	Defect or cavity
Debridement	Removal of foreign material and devitalized or contaminated tissue from a wound until healthy tissue is exposed.
Decubitus	Latin word referring to the reclining position; misnomer for a pressure sore.
Demarcation	Line of separation between viable and nonviable tissue.
Denuded	Loss of epidermis
Disinfectant	Topical liquid chemical that destroys or inhibits growth of microorganisms.
Enzymes	Biochemical substances that are capable of breaking down necrotic tissue.
Epithelialization	Process of the formation of new epithelial tissue-upper layer of the skin.
Erosion	Loss of epidermis
Erythema	Redness of the skin surface produced by vasodilation.
Eschar	Thick, leathery, black or brown crust; can be loose or firmly adherent, hard or soft, dry or wet; it is nonviable tissue and is colonized with bacteria.
Excoriation	Linear scratches on the skin. NOT redness or denuded.
Exudate	Accumulation of fluid in a wound; may contain serum, cellular debris, bacteria, and leukocytes.
Fistula	Abnormal passage from an internal organ to the body surface or between two internal organs.
Friction	Rubbing that causes mechanical trauma to the skin.
Full-thickness	Tissue destruction extending through the dermis to involve subcutaneous level and possibly muscle, fascia, or bone.
Granulation	Formation of connective tissue and many new capillaries in a full-thickness wound; typically appears as red and cobblestoned. Occurs only in a full-thickness wound.

Term	Description
Granulation tissue	The pink to red, moist, fragile capillary tissue that fills a full-thickness wound during the proliferative (cell division) phase of healing.
Hydrophilic	Attracting moisture
Maceration	Softening of tissue by soaking in fluids; looks like "dishpan hands."
MRSA	Methicillin-Resistant *Staphylococcus aureus*
MSSA	Methicillin-Susceptible *Staphylococcus aureus*
Necrotic	Dead; avascular, nonviable
Necrotic tissue	Dead, black or yellow tissue; when soft is referred to as slough, when hard is referred to as eschar.
Occlusive wound dressings	No liquids or gases can be transmitted through the dressing material.
Pallor	Lack of natural color; paleness
Partial-thickness	Wounds that extend through the epidermis and may involve the dermis; these wounds heal by re-epithelialization.
Pus	Thick fluid composed of leukocytes, bacteria, and cellular debris.
Scab	Crust of dried blood and serum.
Semi-occlusive dressing	No liquids are transmitted through dressing naturally; variable level of gases can be transmitted through dressing material; most dressings are semi-occlusive.
Shear	Sliding of skin over subcutaneous tissues and bones, causing a kink in cutaneous capillary that may lead to ischemia.
Sinus tract	A course or pathway which can extend in any direction from the wound base; results in dead space with potential for abscess formation. Also referred to as tunneling.
Skin stripping/Skin tears	The inadvertent removal of the epidermis, with or without the dermis, by mechanical means; precipitated by trauma, such as tape removal, bumping into furniture, or assisting with repositioning.
Slough	Deposits of dead white cells, dead bacteria, etc, in the wound bed, yellow in appearance; soft, moist, avascular/devitalized tissue; may be loose or firmly adherent.
Tunneling	Path of tissue destruction occurring in any direction from the surface or edge of a wound; results in dead space; involves small portion of wound edge; may be referred to as a sinus tract
Undermine	Skin edges of a wound that has lost supporting tissue under intact skin.
VRE	Vancomycin-Resistant *Enterococcus*

Chart content adapted from:

- Bryant RA, Nix DP, eds. *Acute & Chronic Wounds: Current Management Concepts.* 4th ed. St Louis, MO:Elsevier/Mosby. © 2012
- Simonsen H, Coutts P, van den Bogert-Janssen, Knight S. Assessing and managing chronic wounds: wound care reference guide. Coloplast A/S, 2007

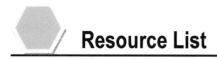

Resource List

BOOKS:

- Burghardt JC, Robinson JM, Tscheschlog BA, Bartelmo JM. *Wound Care Made Incredibly Visual.* 2nd ed. Philadelphia:Lippincott Williams Wilkins © 2012
- Bryant RA, Nix DP, eds. *Acute & Chronic Wounds: Current Management Concepts.* 4th ed. St Louis, MO:Elsevier/Mosby. © 2012
- Hess CT. *Clinical Guide to Skin and Wound Care.* 7th ed. Ambler, PA:Lippincottt, Williams & Wilkins. © 2012

WOUND CARE JOURNALS:

Advances in Skin and Wound Care: http://journals.lww.com/aswcjournal

Advances in Wound Care: http://www.liebertpub.com/overview/advances-in-wound-care

Journal of Wound Care: http://www.journalofwoundcare.com

Ostomy Wound Management: http://www.o-wm.com

Wounds: http://www.woundsresearch.com/wnds

Wounds 360: http://www.wounds360bg.com

MOBILE APPS:

3M Healthcare Pressure Ulcer Staging: no charge; available for Apple/iOS

Cutimed Wound Assessment App: no charge, available for Apple/iOS

Wound Central Mobile App: available for Android or Apple/iOS

ORGANIZATIONS:

Association for the Advancement of Wound Care (AAWC): http://www.aawcone.org

- A multidisciplinary organization with the mission of making wound care better for patients. It is a source of support, information, and education for patients, caregivers, researchers, educators, and practitioners across all settings, including acute, sub-acute, long term care, and at home.

AHRQ: Agency for Healthcare Research and Quality: http://www.ahrq.gov

- AHRQ, a division of the U.S. Department of Health & Human Services, aims to improve the quality, safety, efficiency, and effectiveness of healthcare for all Americans.

BioTherapeutics, Education and Research Foundation (BTER): http://www.bterfoundation.org

- A non-profit organization specializing in public support and professional education in biotherapeutic medicine. Biotherapy is the use of live animals to aid in the diagnosis or treatment of illness.

EPERC: End-of Life/Palliative Education Resource Center: http://www.eperc.mcw.edu

- An end-of-life resource for healthcare professional involved in palliative care through support from the Medical College of Wisconsin.

Hope of Healing Foundation: http://hopeofhealing.org

- Organization founded by physicians to provide community outreach and wound care strategies to prevent amputation

NPUAP-National Pressure Ulcer Advisory Panel: http://www.npuap.org

- American National Pressure Ulcer Advisory Panel: An independent, non-profit professional organization promoting evidence-based care for pressure ulcers.

TOOLS:

- Braden Risk Assessment Scale: Used to assess a patient's risk of developing a pressure ulcer and the degree of risk. It is made up of 6 subscales that contribute to development of pressure ulcers: sensory perception, moisture, activity, mobility, friction and shear. See website for additional information: http://www.bradenscale.com
- Norton Scale: Used to identify patients at-risk for pressure ulcers. There are 5 subscales: physical condition, mental condition, activity, mobility, incontinence. Tool can be found at http://www.ahrq.gov

WEBSITES:

Wound Care Advisor

Official online journal of National Alliance of Wound Care (NAWC) covering wound, skin, and ostomy management

http://woundcareadvisor.com

World Council of Enterstomal Therapists

Association for nurses involved in ostomy, wound, and continence care

http://www.wcetn.org

Wound Ostomy and Continence Nurses Society

Nursing society supporting educational, clinical, and research opportunities in an effort to guide the delivery of health care to individuals with wounds, ostomies, and incontinence. *Photography in Wound Documentation: Fact Sheet* available via the WOCN website.

http://www.wocn.org

Ostomy Wound Management

Journal for health care professionals addressing ostomy care, wound care, incontinence care, and related skin and nutritional issues. Includes Wounds 360 online wound care products resource

http://www.o-wm.com

WoundSource.com

Provides wound care professionals clinically-reviewed, wound care supplies information. Includes over 1,000 products manufactured by over 150 wound care companies

http://www.WoundSource.com

WorldWideWounds.com

Web-based wound care journal covering dressing materials and wound management topics

http://www.WorldWideWounds.com

CUMULATIVE REFERENCE LIST

- Agency for Health Care Policy and Research (AHCPR). *Pressure ulcers in adults: prediction and prevention*. Clinical Practice Guideline no.3; AHCPR-92-0047, May 1992. [Internet] Available from: http://www.eric.ed.gov/PDFS/ED357247.pdf. Accessed 6/6/2012

- Alvarez OM, Kalinski C, Nusbaum J, Hernandez L, Pappous E, Kyriannis C, et al. Incorporating wound healing strategies to improve palliation (symptom management) in patients with chronic wounds. *J Palliat Med* 2007;10(5):1161-1189

- Alvarez OM, Meehan M, Ennis W, Thomas DR, Ferris FD, Kennedy KL, Rogers , et al. Chronic wounds: palliative management for the frail population, parts 1-4, *Wounds* 2002;14(10)

- American Association for Long Term Care Nursing (AALTCN). Ask the Wound Coach. [Internet] Available from: http://ltcnursing.org/ask-the-wound-coach.htm. Accessed 6/6/2012

- Ayello EA, Capitulo KL, Fowler E, Krasner DL, Mulder G, Sibbald RG, Yankowsky KW. Legal issues in the care of pressure ulcer patients: key concepts for health care providers: a consensus paper from the International Expert Wound Care Advisory Panel. *J Palliat Med* 2009;12(11):995-1008

- Baharvand M, Sarrafi M, Alavi K, Jalali ME. Efficacy of topical phenytoin on chemotherapy-induced oral mucositis: a pilot study. *DARU* 2010;18(1):46-50

- Broderick N. Understanding chronic wound healing. *Nurse Practitioner* 2009;34(10):16-22

- Brown G. Wound documentation: managing risk. *Adv Skin Wound Care* 2006;19(3):155-165

- Brown P. *Quick reference to wound care*. 4th ed. Burlington, MA: Jones & Bartlett Learning; c2012. Chapter 4 Basics of wound management; p. 25-40

- Bryant RA. Types of skin damage and differential diagnosis. In Bryant RA, Nix DP, eds. *Acute & Chronic Wounds: Current Management Concepts.* 4th ed. St Louis, MO:Elsevier/Mosby. © 2012, p83-107

- Collins N. The facts about vitamin C and wound healing. *Ostomy Wound Manage* 2009;55(3):8-9

- Cutting KF. Honey and contemporary wound care: an overview. *Ostomy Wound Manage* 2007;53(11):49-54

- Doughty DB, Sparks-DeFriese B. Wound-healing physiology. In Bryant RA, Nix DP, eds. *Acute & Chronic Wounds: Current Management Concepts.* 4th ed. St Louis, MO:Elsevier/Mosby. © 2012, p63-82

- Doughty DB. Arterial ulcers. In Bryant RA, Nix DP, eds. *Acute & Chronic Wounds: Current Management Concepts.* 4th ed. St Louis, MO:Elsevier/Mosby. © 2012, p178-193

- Drosou A, Falabella A, Kirsner RS. Antiseptics on wounds: an area of controversy. Wounds 2008. [Internet] Available from: http://www.woundsresearch.com/article/1586

- Enoch S, Price P. Cellular, molecular and biochemical differences in the pathophysiology of healing between acute wounds, chronic wounds and wounds in the aged, August 2004. Available at http://www.worldwidewounds.com/2004/august/Enoch/Pathophysiology-Of-Healing.html. Accessed 6/6/2012

- Enoch S, Shaaban H, Dunn KW. Informed consent should be obtained from patients to use products (skin substitutes) and dressings containing biological material. *J Med Ethics* 2005;31:2-6

- Ermer-Selton J. Lower extremity assessment. In Bryant RA, Nix DP, eds. *Acute & Chronic Wounds: Current Management Concepts.* 4th ed. St Louis, MO:Elsevier/Mosby. © 2012, p169-177

- Evans E, Gray M. Do topical analgesics reduce pain associated with wound dressing changes or debridement of chronic wounds? *J Wound Ostomy Continence Nurs* 2005;32(5):287-290

- Fogh K, Glynn C, Junger M, Krasner DL, Price P, Sibbald RG. Assessing and managing painful chronic wounds: a pocket guide. Coloplast A/S, 2007. [Internet] Available from: http://www.coloplast.com/WoundAndSkinCare/Topics/WoundManagement/Documents/Assessing%20and%20Managing%20Painful%20Chronic%20Wounds.pdf Accessed 6/6/2012

- Gammaitoni A, Gallagher R, Welz-Bozna M. Topical ketamine gel:possible role in treating neuropathic pain. *Pain Med* 2000;1(1):97-100

- Gestring M, Sanfey H, Collins KA. Negative pressure wound therapy. In UpToDate, Basow DS ed. Waltham, MA. 2012

- Goldberg MT, Bryant RA. Managing wounds in palliative care. In Bryant RA, Nix DP, eds. *Acute & Chronic Wounds: Current Management Concepts.* 4th ed. St Louis, MO:Elsevier/Mosby. © 2012, p505-513

- Hess CT. Managing tissue loads. *Adv Skin Wound Care* 2008;21(3):144

- Hess CT. The art of skin and wound care. *Home Healthcare Nurse* 2005;23(8):502-513

- Hess CT. Understanding the barriers to healing. *Adv Skin Wound Care* 2012;25(5):240

- Hinshaw J. Larval therapy: a review of clinical human and veterinary studies. October 2000. [Internet] Available from: http://www.worldwidewounds.com/2000/oct/Janet-Hinshaw/Larval-Therapy-Human-and-Veterinary.html. Accessed 6/6/2012

- Hopf HW, Shapshak D, Junkins S. Managing wound pain. In Bryant RA, Nix DP, eds. *Acute & Chronic Wounds: Current Management Concepts.* 4th ed. St Louis, MO:Elsevier/Mosby. © 2012, p380-387

- Institute for Clinical Systems Improvement (ICSI). *Health Care Protocol: Skin safety protocol: risk assessment and prevention of pressure ulcers.* March 2007. [Internet] Available from: http://www.njha.com/qualityinstitute/pdf/226200833420PM63.pdf. Accessed 6/6/2012

- Jacobson J. Topical opioids for pain. *Fast Facts and Concepts* 2007; 184. [Internet] Available from: http://www.eperc.mcw.edu/fastfact/ff_184.htm

- Kalinski C, Schnepf M, Laboy D, Hernandez L, Nusbaum J, McGrinder B, Alvarez OM. Effectiveness of a topical formulation containing metronidazole for wound odor and exudate control. *Wounds* 2005;17(5):84-90

- Karukonda SRK, Flynn TC, Boh EE, McBurney EI, Russo GG, Millikan LE. The effects of drugs on wound healing- part II. Specific classes of drugs and their effect on healing wounds. *Int J Dermatol* 2000;39:321-333

- Kelechi TJ, Johnson JJ. Guideline for the management of wounds in patients with lower-extremity venous disease: an executive summary. *J Wound Ostomy Continence Nurs* 2012;39(6):598-606

- Kennedy-Evans K. Understanding the Kennedy terminal ulcer. *Ostomy Wound Manage* 2009;55(9):6

- Krasner DL, Rodeheaver GT, Sibbald RG. Interprofessional wound caring. In Krasner DL, Rodeheaver GT, Sibbald RG, eds *Chronic Wound Care: A Clinical Sourcebook for Healthcare Professionals.* 4th ed. Malvern, PA: HMP Communications. ©2007, p.3-9

- Langemo D. General principles and approaches to wound prevention and care at the end of life: an overview. *Ostomy Wound Manage* 2012;58(5):24-34

- LeBlanc K, Baranoski S, Skin Tear Consensus Panel Members. Skin tears: state of the science: consensus statements for the prevention, prediction, assessment, and treatment of skin tears. *Adv Skin Wound Care* 2012;24(9suppl):2-15

- Lexi-Comp Online, Lexi-Drugs Online, Hudson, Ohio: Lexi-Comp, Inc.; June 6, 2012

- Lippincott, Williams and Wilkins. *Wound Care Made Incredibly Visual.* 2nd Edition

- Lyder CH, Ayello EA. Pressure ulcers: a patient safety issue. In Agency for Healthcare Research and Quality. *Patient Safety and Quality: An Evidence-Based Handbook for Nurses.* AHRQ Pub No. 08-0043, April 2008. [Internet] Available from: http://www.ahrq.gov/qual/nurseshdbk/docs/lyderc_pupsi.pdf. Accessed 6/6/2012

- Lynch M, Clark A, Sawynok J, Sullivan M. Topical 2% amitriptyline and 1% ketamine in neuropathic pain syndromes. *Anesthesiology* 2005;103:140-6

- Mahoney J, Vardaxis V, Moore J, Hall A, Haffner K, Peterson M. Topical ketamine cream in the treatment of diabetic peripheral neuropathy. *J Am Podiatr Med Assoc* 2012;102(3):178-183

- McDonald A, Lesage P. Palliative management of pressure ulcers and malignant wounds in patients with advanced illness. *J Palliat Med* 2005;9(2):285-295

- Moffat S. Understanding compression therapy. 2003; Medical Education Partnership LTD, 2003; European Wound Management Association (EWMA). [Internet] Available from: http://www.woundsinternational.com/pdf/content_51.pdf

- Molan PC. Honey as topical antibacterial agent for treatment of infected wounds. December 2001. Available at http://www.worldwidewounds.com/2001/november/Molan/honey-as-topical-agent.html. Accessed 6/6/2012

- National Pressure Ulcer Advisory Panel (NPUAP-EPUAP). Updated staging system: pressure ulcer stages revised by NPUAP. February 2007. [Internet] Available from: http://npuap.org/pr2.htm. Accessed 6/6/2012

- National Pressure Ulcer Advisory Panel (NPUAP-EPUAP).Pressure Ulcer Prevention and Treatment Guidelines. October 2009

- National Pressure Ulcer Advisory Panel. NPUAP White Paper [Internet]. Deep tissue injury. 2012. [Internet] Available from: http://www.npuap.org/wp-content/uploads/2012/01/DTI-White-Paper.pdf

- Netsch DS. Negative pressure wound therapy. In Bryant RA, Nix DP, eds. *Acute & Chronic Wounds: Current Management Concepts.* 4th ed. St Louis, MO:Elsevier/Mosby. © 2012, p337-344

- Nix DP, Peirce B. Noncompliance, nonadherence, or barriers to a sustainable plan? In Bryant RA, Nix DP, eds. *Acute & Chronic Wounds: Current Management Concepts.* 4th ed. St Louis, MO:Elsevier/Mosby. © 2012, p408-415

- O'Meara S, Cullum NA, Nelson EA. Compression for venous leg ulcers. *Cochrane Database Syst Rev* 2009; 29(1):CD000265

- Patel B, Cox-Hayley D. Managing wound odor. *Fast Facts & Concepts.* August 2009; 218. Available at http://www.eperc.mcw.edu/EPERC/FastFactsIndex/ff_218.htm. Accessed 6/6/2012

- Pieper B. Pressure ulcers: impact, etiology, and classification. In Bryant RA, Nix DP, eds. *Acute & Chronic Wounds: Current Management Concepts.* 4th ed. St Louis, MO:Elsevier/Mosby. © 2012, p123-136

- Pontani B, Feste M, Adams C, et al. Cross over clinical study of 47 patients with painful deep wounds showed use of a hydrogel containing 2% lidocaine HCl and collagen as contact layer was significant in alleviating dressing related pain. 23rd Clinical Symposium on Advances in Skin & Wound Care Oct 2008, no.30.

- Popescu A, Salcido R. Wound pain: a challenge for the patient and the wound care specialist. *Adv Skin Wound Care* 2004;17:14-22
- Posthauer ME. Does zinc supplementation accelerate wound healing? [Internet] Available from: http://www.woundsource.com/blog/does-zinc-supplementation-accelerate-wound-healing Accessed 11/30/2012
- Posthauer ME. Palliative care challenges: offering supportive nutritional care at end of life. [Internet] Available from: http://www.woundsource.com/blog/palliative-care-challenges-offering-supportive-nutritional-care-end-life. Accessed 6/6/2012
- Quan D, Wellish M, Gilden D. Topical ketamine treatment of postherpetic neuralgia. *Neurology* 2003;60(8):1391-2
- Quibell R, Prommer E, Mihalyo M, Twycross R, Wilcock A. Ketamine: therapeutic review. *J Pain Symptom Manage* 2011;41(3):640-649
- Ramundo J. Wound debridement. In Bryant RA, Nix DP, eds. *Acute & Chronic Wounds: Current Management Concepts.* 4th ed. St Louis, MO:Elsevier/Mosby. © 2012, p279-288
- Ratliff CR. WOCN's evidence-based pressure ulcer guidelines. *Adv Skin Wound Care* 2005;18(4):204-208
- Rolstad BS, Bryant RA, Nix DP. Topical management. In Bryant RA, Nix DP, eds. *Acute & Chronic Wounds: Current Management Concepts.* 4th ed. St Louis, MO:Elsevier/Mosby. © 2012, p289-306
- Ryan A, Lin F, Atayee R. Ketamine mouthwash for mucositis pain. *J Palliat Med* 2009;12(11);989-91
- Santos PW, Hartle JE, Quarles LD. Calciphylaxis. In UpToDate, Goldfarb S. (Ed) UpToDate, Waltham, MA, 2012
- Shaw J, Hughes CM, Lagan KM, Bell PM. The clinical effect of topical phenytoin on wound healing: a systematic review. *Brit J Dermatol* 2007;157:997-1004
- Shaw J, Hughes CM, Lagan KM, Stevenson MR, Irwin CR, Bell PM. The effect of topical phenytoin on healing diabetic foot ulcers: a randomized controlled trial. *Diabet Med* 2011;28:1154-1157
- Sherman RA, Pechter EA. Maggot therapy: a review of the therapeutic applications of fly larvae in human medicine, especially for treating osteomyelitis. *Med Vet Entomology* 1988;2(3):225-230
- Sibbald RG, Krasner DL, Lutz J. SCALE: Skin changes at life's end: final consensus statement: October 1, 2009. *Adv Skin Wound Care* 2010;23(5):225-236
- Sibbald RG, Woo K, Ayello EA. Increased bacterial burden and infection: the story of NERDS and STONES. *Adv Skin Wound Care* 2006;19(8):447-461
- Simonsen H, Coutts P, van den Bogert-Janssen, Knight S. Assessing and managing chronic wounds: wound care reference guide. Coloplast A/S, 2007. [Internet] Available from: http://www.coloplast.com/woundandskincare/topics/woundmanagement/woundassessment/woundcarerefguide. Accessed 6/6/2012
- Slatkin N, Rhiner M. Topical ketamine in the treatment of mucositis pain. *Pain Med* 2004;4(3):298-303
- Song JJ, Salcido R. Use of honey in wound care: an update. *Adv Skin Wound Care* 2011;24(1):40-44
- Spahn J. Support surfaces: science and practice. Presented at First Annual Palliative Wound Care Conference, May 13-14, 2010. Hope of Healing Foundation. Cincinnati, Ohio

- Stotts N. Nutritional assessment and support. In Bryant RA, Nix DP, eds. *Acute & Chronic Wounds: Current Management Concepts.* 4th ed. St Louis, MO:Elsevier/Mosby. © 2012, p388-399

- Stotts N. Wound infection: diagnosis and management. In Bryant RA, Nix DP, eds. *Acute & Chronic Wounds: Current Management Concepts.* 4th ed. St Louis, MO:Elsevier/Mosby. © 2012, p270-278

- Teno J, Gozalo P, Mitchell SL, Kuo S, Fulton AT, Mor V. Feeding tubes and the prevention or healing of pressure ulcers. *Arch Intern Med* 2012;172(9):697-701

- Tippett A. How does biotherapy relate to wound care? WoundSource.com. January 2012. [Internet] Available from: http://www.woundsource.com/blog/how-does-biotherapy-relate-wound-care. Accessed 6/6/2012

- Tran QNH, Fancher T. Achieving analgesia for painful ulcers using topically applied morphine gel. *J Support Oncol* 2007;5(6):289-293

- Whitney JD. Perfusion and oxygenation. In Bryant RA, Nix DP, eds. *Acute & Chronic Wounds: Current Management Concepts.* 4th ed. St Louis, MO:Elsevier/Mosby. © 2012, p400-407

- Woo KY, Sibbald RG. Local wound care for malignant and palliative wounds. *Adv Skin Wound Care.* 2010;23(9):417-428

- Wound Union of Wound Healing Societies (WUWHS). Woundpedia: evidence informed practice: Ostomy/Continence/Skin Care. [Internet] Available from: http://www.woundpedia.com/ Accessed 6/6/2012

- Zeppetella G, Joel SP, Ribeiro MDC. Stability of morphine sulphate and diamorphine hydrochloride in Intrasite gel. *Palliat Med* 2005;19:131-136

- Zip CM. Innovative use of topical metronidazole. *Dermatol Clin* 2010;28(3):525-534

Index

Made in the USA
San Bernardino, CA
07 September 2014